Evidence-Based Chiropractic Care for Infants

Rationale, Therapies, and Outcomes

Joyce Miller, DC, PhD

Praeclarus Press, LLC

www.PraeclarusPress.com

Praeclarus Press, LLC

2504 Sweetgum Lane

Amarillo, Texas 79124 USA

806-367-9950

www.PraeclarusPress.com

DISCLAIMER

The information contained in this publication is advisory only and is not intended to replace sound clinical judgment or individualized patient care. The author disclaims all warranties, whether expressed or implied, including any warranty as the quality, accuracy, safety, or suitability of this information for any particular purpose.

ISBN: 978-1-946665-36-2

Cover Design: Ken Tackett

Developmental Editing: Kathleen Kendall-Tackett

Copyediting: Chris Tackett

Layout & Design: Nelly Murariu

Contents

CHAPTER 1

Why Evidence Is Necessary for Infant Healthcare

All healthcare professionals are focused on providing the best possible care for each patient. But what is the best type of care? Answering that question is where evidence becomes important. What is most effective? What doesn't work? Clinicians cannot rely just upon their own experience (although that is an important factor to guide care) but must also look into what types of care researchers have tested, and whether these types of care benefitted the infant and family. Therefore, the focus of this small book is to investigate, describe, and explain the types of conservative care for newborns and infants that chiropractors and other manual-therapy professionals have done, and to delineate the results and what those results mean for the parent, clinician, and patient. All of this is grounded, not only in opinion, but in evidence provided by specific studies designed to answer research questions. The main focus herein is on chiropractic care (comprised for infants largely as manual therapy), partly because that is my main interest, but also because it is the most commonly used type of care for infants outside of medicine (Black et al., 2015; Kemper et al., 2008). Among pediatric patients, infants are overrepresented in the chiropractors' office, comprising at least two-thirds of their pediatric practice (Hestbaek, Jorgensen, & Hartvigsen, 2009; Miller, 2010).

Medical care is the mainstay for healthcare in families who require urgent or illness care, as that is usually considered crisis care and is the best care for those types of conditions. Through the ages, there has been consistent research done in these areas, though too little in the infant population. The reason for too little evidence is that infants are a vulnerable group, and it can be difficult to get ethical approval for research. When researching drugs and surgery, there are high risks to the well-being of the infant and concerns about the side effects of these types of care (Conroy et al., 2000). However, most infants require well-baby care; care that is not crisis-oriented, but rather, quality-of-life oriented. Chiropractors are the most common provider of this type of care for infants, outside of the medical profession. This care is called conservative. Chiropractic care for infants also has too little evidence, but there is a growing body of research that is the focus of this book.

The purpose of this book is to provide to the clinician, chiropractor, family, or parents a description of some of the key research on conservative clinical care for the infant. All of this is available elsewhere, as this work is based on published studies. I've included these studies in the reference section for ease of access. This work is designed to put much of the information in one place to make it easily accessible, in plain English, to save time in understanding. Anyone requiring further details can use the references for their research. It is best to read the original work and form your own opinion, rather than rely on mine. As an author, I am completely biased. My life's goal is to increase the respect that all humanity has for the infant and, most particularly, for the infant patient who may be experiencing pain or problems. I feel that conservative therapy with skilled hands is a way forward to honor the infant and treat those with biomechanical irritants safely. There is very little risk for even mild side effects, and there is strong evidence for a good result and very high parent satisfaction.

What is Chiropractic Care?

Chiropractic care is manual medicine and is one of the most common types of manual therapies, which include osteopathy, physiotherapy, and other lay or professional therapies. Chiropractors are musculoskeletalists who differ from most other types of manual therapists in that chiropractors are trained as primary contact clinicians with diagnostic training. They have extensive knowledge of specific types of manual therapies (WHO, 2005). As such, it is a profession that dedicates itself to the prevention and treatment of musculoskeletal problems for humans of all ages. Chiropractors perform about 96% of the manual therapy provided to patients in the world today. The World Health Organization (2005) defines chiropractic care as:

> A health care profession concerned with the diagnosis, treatment and prevention of disorders of the neuromusculoskeletal system and the effects of these disorders on general health.

The chiropractic profession has been in existence for over 100 years and is the third largest healthcare profession in the world, after general medical practice and dentistry (Mootz, Hansen, Breen, Killinger, & Nelson, 2006). Chiropractors focus upon mechanical stress of the human body, and this begins from the time of intrauterine life and includes passage through the birth canal (Stellwagen, Hubbard, Chambers, & Lyons-Jones, 2008). It also includes everyday life stresses, which can manifest as pain, loss of function, and even disability (Nyiendo, Haas, & Hondras, 1997).

Chiropractic therapy is demarcated by the use of manual manipulation of joints and soft tissues intended to promote the health and well-being of the patient. It may encompass a wide variety of techniques or modalities, including manipulative therapy, light touch (touch and hold, or hold and release), moderate touch or deeper pressure involving treatment of trigger points, myofascial release, neuromuscular techniques, or massage to the soft tissues, and nutritional and wellness advice.

Touch is the first sense to develop in humans, and therapeutic touch therapy has been known and used in healthcare since the time of Hippocrates (c. 460 BC to 370 BC). Touch continues in use for pain control in modern medicine for even premature neonates, where it has been found to be very beneficial (Honda et al., 2013). Significant benefits of chiropractic manual therapy for pain control in adults have been documented in many analyses (Moyer, Rounds, & Hannum, 2004).

Why Would a Newborn Need Chiropractic Care?

In pediatric patients, it is the youngest group who present to chiropractors most commonly (Hestbaek et al., 2009; Miller, 2010). At first glance, it may not seem plausible that they require care. There has been so little time for the newborn to sustain a mechanical injury, like a sprain or strain, the types of common injuries presented to chiropractors. What is relevant, and often implicated, is the birth history, along with any prenatal history of constraint. Chiropractors treat musculoskeletal and biomechanical conditions, usually described as imbalances. These can commonly occur either before birth or during birth, in what has been termed physiologic birth injury (PBI) (Rabello, Matushita, & Cardeal, 2017). This is the term that we can all adopt to focus on the potential musculoskeletal injuries that may affect the newborn. It is a more clinically useful term than birth trauma, which has a much wider definition and can affect both mother and baby. The mother may also require care, but this book concentrates on the specific difficulties of the baby.

More boys than girls are presented at the earliest age. This may be at least partly because more boys than girls are conceived and born. However, the more likely reason may be that the slightly larger boys may have had more intrauterine constraint before birth, and more difficulty traveling through the birth canal because of their size. It has been well-documented that infants presented to chiropractors have high incidence of assisted or interventional births (Miller, Beharie, Taylor, Simmenes, & Way, 2016). It is also well-documented that more birth injuries occur with interventions (Kozak & Weeks, 2002). For many years, infants assessed at birth, or presented to clinics with pain, have demonstrated mechanical strains and restrictions, or notable birth trauma (Edwards, Gibb, & Cook, 2010; Frymann, 1966). It is no surprise that musculoskeletal irritation is present at all ages (Miller, 2013). Those most at risk in the earliest ages are male babies, born of primiparous (first-time) mothers with medical interventions (Levine et al., 1984; Torvaldson, Roberts, Simpson, Thompson, & Elwood, 2006).

Few professions are trained in the management of musculoskeletal issues of infants. Research suggests that medical doctors have more concerns about life-and-death issues and little education on the biomechanics of the child (Jandial, Myers, & Wise, 2009). It is logical that a profession that focuses on the life and death of the newborn would have little interest in biomechanics and joints, issues that can cause profound quality-of-life problems but seldom include life-threatening injuries or death.

Chiropractors have the education and background to provide conservative care for the newborn's issues that may stem from a difficult birth history. But this care, like any healthcare, needs to develop an evidence base as to whether or not it is effective, safe, or even cost-effective. These studies have been done and will be discussed. More studies are needed as well. But first, it is important to understand what mothers want from this type of healthcare. She has experienced the birth, often with great discomfort. What an understatement!

Birth Can be Difficult

Many healthcare professionals may suspect that birth injuries are rare when obstetric standards are high. The effects of assisted and instrumental births are often ignored, or the injuries caused may be overlooked (the baby cannot point to any pain or irritation). A mother may feel very alone and may find that few are interested in hearing stories about her difficult birth. She may minimize the problems once she sees the beautiful product of birth: the baby.

Birth has been described as "the most difficult trip that a human being ever takes" (unknown source). Birth trauma is a difficult concept because everyone's perception is different. Medicine may suggest that there is no trauma unless the baby is dead or brain-damaged. The father may be reluctant to talk about it. The mother may have a range of issues regarding the birth, from denial to sheer terror, as she discusses it. We must look at the mechanism to understand what the baby has been through. It must be kept in mind that in this scenario, the baby is our patient, not the parents, although their experience is clearly relevant.

Routine birth is a blend of compression, contractions, torques, and traction. Even a "normal delivery presents a trauma to the infant"

(Rabelo, Matushita, & Cardeal, 2017). Medicine quickly investigates hypoxia and neurological damage: life and death stuff. Chiropractors investigate compressions, strains, and pain: quality-of-life stuff. When mothers ask us why their doctor did not see the imbalances, we can explain it in that way. These babies are often sent to us (chiropractors) right from the hospital.

Some authors suggest that birth may be traumatic for the baby and unavoidable, and recommend evaluation immediately after birth to detect problems early to avoid long-term consequences, such as chronic pain syndromes (Stellwagen et al., 2008).

There are many causes of physiologic birth injury to the newborn. One cause may be precipitate labor or rapid labor that occurs in under three hours. Mother's tissues need time to adapt, and the baby's head needs time to compress, and neither of these may occur successfully if the birth is too rapid.

Intrauterine position and posture are important as well. It has long been known that there is significant long-term effect (up to 18 months of age) in infants born after uncomplicated breech position compared with control infants (Sival, Prechtl, Sonder, & Touwen, 1993). Musculoskeletal monitoring in the long-term is the right approach for these children.

In a large practice of chiropractors treating infants in the UK, there was over-representation of assisted births in practice (Miller et al., 2009-2018). Routinely, about 32% of births in any local UK hospital (that manages all types of births) require assistance. In chiropractic practice, the rate is much higher, at least double, depending on the study. Furthermore, it must be kept in mind that even a "natural, unassisted birth can be a traumatic experience for the infant, and much can happen in utero prior to delivery" (Gottlieb, 1993).

Graph showing more common birth interventions reported in infants presented by their parents to a clinic in the UK.

We can expect that "small" injuries, where there is little insult that shows on the surface of the tissue, may be missed. There may be only bruises or abrasions. However, there may also be occult impairments in the dynamic mobility of the articulations (joints) often called fixations or blockages of the musculoskeletal system. These problems are difficult to find, as they are not likely to show on X-ray or ultrasound, nor would anyone routinely consider imaging the baby, as that could be harmful in and of itself. But chiropractors can locate musculoskeletal alterations through skilled palpation. The point is to remove the imbalances in the joints and soft tissues, thus restoring normal movement patterns. This book is precisely about how these kinds of injuries present in the infant and what the methods are, and the evidence for their treatment.

Many believe that birth injury is rare. This is true for severe injury, but mild-to-moderate injuries are common. Babies often present, for example, with clavicle fractures (see photo). These will heal on their own, but we can tape them to improve the comfort of the baby.

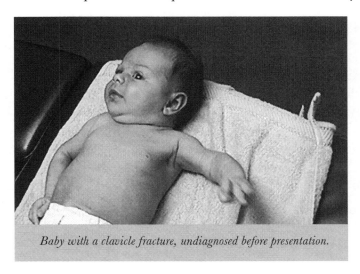

Baby with a clavicle fracture, undiagnosed before presentation.

Why Are We Concerned about the Musculoskeletal Health of Infants?

Despite musculoskeletal disorders being the leading cause of pain, and the second greatest cause of disability around the world today, according to the World Health Organization (WHO; World Health Organization, 2012), the musculoskeletal health of infants has been inadequately studied. Musculoskeletal maladaptation in infants is defined here as a failure of the motor system to respond or to respond, correctly, to appropriate sensory stimuli due to biomechanical fault (Ferreira & James, 1972; Prechtl et al., 1997; Reher, Kuny, Pantalitchka, Urschitz, & Poets, 2008). In other words, the brain calls for action, but the body is unable to respond appropriately.

Normal response patterns are generated when the musculoskeletal system responds appropriately to the central nervous system that mediates sensorimotor integration of the environmental and physiological demands. When the musculoskeletal system cannot respond to normal signals due to biomechanical compromise, then the infant's response to signals may be inappropriate, inefficient, ineffective or aberrant, or even uncomfortable or painful. These responses become characterized as functional problems of infancy and most commonly include excessive crying, inefficient sleep habits, and sometimes ineffective feeding (St. James-Roberts, 2008). Parents usually seek help for these and other problems of infancy. However, they are often termed "medically unexplained symptoms." That is probably due to a lack of understanding rather than from lacking a clear explanation, which usually is quite apparent.

Little is known about the impact of musculoskeletal dysfunctions in infancy other than that they account for significant use of resources. While half the expenditure on adult healthcare can be attributed to musculoskeletal disorders (WHO, 2012), the cost in infancy is also high. Morris and colleagues (2001) calculated the cost of infant crying and sleeping problems as £65 million to the National Health Service in the UK during the first 12 weeks of life, with no evidence of benefit to the child. There are many indirect costs among parents and family members as well, including maternal depression, exhaustion, lost time at work, and marital disharmony (Bromfield & Holzer, 2008). These costs were recalculated in 2015 and found to be over £186 million ($306 million) (Miller, 2013). This is a great deal of money spent that shows no benefit, and this was only for the problems of crying and sleeping in infants. It begs us to question, what do mothers want from healthcare for their newborn? We decided to ask them.

CHAPTER 2

What Do Mothers Want from Healthcare for their Newborn?

A ll healthcare professionals strive to provide patient-centered care. But can we be sure what this is without asking? We decided to ask mothers of newborn babies what they wanted from the healthcare for their newborn (Miller et al., 2015). This study is described here and served as a basis for further patient-outcomes research.

Picture five young researchers setting out with a goal to provide for infant healthcare what has been done for all other age groups: to develop Patient Reported Outcomes Measures (PROMs). This type of survey has been increasingly advocated as a means of supporting patient-centered care, informing better healthcare decisions, and improving quality of service (Bodger, Ormerod, Shackcloth, & Harrison, 2014). It has been stressed that the best way to assure that the content of these surveys is suitable to the patient being studied is to ask them, as this assures what is called content validity (the questionnaire measures what it was intended to measure) (Bredart, Marrel, & Abetz-Webb, 2014).

This all sounds great from a desire to improve healthcare. The problem is whether this approach would work with a very sensitive, fatigued, and overwhelmed group, who are not even the patient but the mothers of the patients. Further, this step requires what is called qualitative research, which can be quite difficult to manage, as it takes a great deal of one-to-one time with the mother of a new baby, who most certainly has far better things to do than sit for an interview. Undaunted, the young researchers devised a plan, submitted it for ethical review, which it passed with much scrutiny just because it is such a vulnerable group of parents, and then asked mothers to participate.

The father's experience of the birth of a preterm infant had been previously investigated (Lundquist, Hellstrom-Westas, & Hellstrom, 2014), but the mother's experience of healthcare for the healthy infant has received too little focus. Mothers who presented to the clinic signed consent and were interviewed, either one-on-one or in a focus group: whichever they chose. Questions were wide-ranging, and mothers could present their own topic of conversation, should they choose. This is both the value and the challenge of qualitative research: that it is guided as much by the person being interviewed as the interviewer. Hence, this is considered the best way to find out what is really on the mother's mind and does not restrict her to specific topics. We were concerned that new mothers would not wish to participate.

However, participate they did. It turned out that our concern that mothers would not have time or interest to participate were soon alleviated, as mothers quickly volunteered. In all, 34 mothers participated, far more than is usually required for such research. After 12 interviews, the information gathered is generally considered saturated, without new information surfacing (Brod, Tesler, & Christensen, 2009). We used more than double the number recommended, as we did not want to miss any idea that mothers would provide about what they want from healthcare. The published study can be read in *Clinical Lactation* (Miller et al., 2015).

What do mothers want? In a nutshell, they valued honest and realistic reassurance. That means that they don't want to be told, "there, there, it will be alright." They want to be told exactly why their baby suffers. For example, when the problem is breastfeeding, they want to be told why the baby has difficulty attaching to the breast, difficulty transferring milk, etc., and NOT that it will probably be okay in the end. They want to know specifics about their baby, when it is a problem with the baby, and when it is a problem with the mother (seldom, but the mother tends to think she is always at fault).

They often stated that they were very grateful that they had been referred to a chiropractor because they were getting straight answers to their questions, a good analysis of the baby's problem, and were not brushed aside, but taken as seriously as the problem is. They want to know what can be done, if anything, and how long it will take. They were concerned about the amount of conflicting advice that they had received along the way. But what they wanted most was to be truly listened to by the professional. They had concerns about their baby (see Box below).

> *Mothers' concerns for their babies as given during interviews, in their own words.*
>
> » Pain
>
> » Difficulty breastfeeding
>
> » Difficulty finding comfort in sleeping on their back
>
> » Excessive irritability or crying
>
> » Distorted head shape
>
> » Refusal to do tummy time
>
> » Sleep periods too short or too restless for the age of the baby
>
> » Difficulty in turning head side to side or other movement patterns, or difficulty feeding on one side
>
> » Mothers felt anxiety or depression about their baby's problems and felt that their quality of life had deteriorated

The mothers' concerns then became topics for the questionnaire that was under development so that further study could be done to find out whether clinicians can help with these problems. Mothers often related the need for chiropractic care to birth interventions. This was the key reason that their babies had been sent to our office by their midwife, GP, health visitor, or pediatrician. Mothers talked freely and extensively about the birth. Sometimes we noted that this seemed to be the first time that they had had a chance to unload the difficulties and details of the birth. There was a great diversity in the type and amount of support that the mothers had received from different healthcare professionals. They were very pleased that those professionals, who did not feel that they could help, referred onward for chiropractic care. This is a hallmark of patient-centered care. If other care is required in our practices, those mothers are referred elsewhere.

Mothers felt physically and emotionally fatigued. They protected the rest of the family from these exact issues, and they bore the brunt of caring for the baby 24 hours a day. Their exhaustion was amplified when babies had difficulty lying comfortably on their back, so mothers felt that they had to be held all the time. This is a public health issue, as supine sleep is required to lower the risk for Sudden Infant Death Syndrome (SIDS) and is emphasized in the Back-To-Sleep program (AAP, 1992, 2016). This is a clear indication of the need for manual therapy. Chiropractic care is a key treatment approach for those babies who cannot sleep comfortably on their backs (Miller et al., 2018; Schmid et al., 2016; Wright et al., 2014). All healthcare professionals must remain vigilant to recognize these cases and get help.

The mothers' points-of-view were invaluable in creating a patient-centered survey dedicated to the infant patient. The next step was to develop and validate the survey for wider usage.

CHAPTER 3

Making Sure That the Survey Is Accurate, Valid, and Reliable

First, why not use an existing survey? Did we have to re-invent the wheel? Researchers have been concerned about the common problems of infants for a very long time, at least 70 years, when the term infant colic was coined to describe the crying baby who appeared to be experiencing significant pain (Wessel, Cobb, Jackson, Harris, & Detwilter, 1954). It is true that there are surveys that assess routine infant problems (crying, sleeping, and feeding). The situation is that each survey only assesses a single problem. What mothers told us is that the baby will often demonstrate more than one issue, sometimes several in a "package." Researchers, likewise, stated that these problems often co-exist (Hemmi, Wolke, & Schneider, 2011). That team also found that these problems, when found in infancy, could have long-term sequelae as well. This was another and very valid reason to work toward a good outcomes instrument to determine whether healthcare helped these infants' maladies or not. It is always important to strive to prevent long-term problems.

A survey can be especially helpful for physically and emotionally exhausted mothers who are worried about their babies and want to be sure to include all the problems, not just the most obvious one. Surveys like this shine over simple interviews because no information is left behind. Further, it is a direct report from the mother before she has even met with the clinician, so her observations have been found to be very objective and very accurate, particularly because there has, as yet, been no subjective interpretation by the clinician (Bredart, Marrel, & Abetz-Webb, 2014).

Despite the importance of listening to the child and parents, which was advocated by the NHS Care Quality Commission (2015), this type of research has never been developed for this age group in this setting, not least because of age restrictions and ethical concerns. Another issue is the very long and tedious process of determining what is important for mothers to survey, working through a process of validation, and assessing whether the form is, in fact, reliable. Hence, a two-plus year process began to develop what came to be called the United Kingdom Infant Questionnaire (UKIQ). The thought was that if all of the work came to fruition, it might answer critics regarding lack of research (Ernst, 2009) because this survey might be used in research if it proved to be valid.

There were seven phases to the research, which can be viewed in both the M-level dissertation (where the methods required a full 36 pages to describe), along with the publication that reveals a shorter form of the process (Miller et al., 2016). It was a complicated process because each question needed to be validated separately (because there were no previously validated full forms) and it had to be shown to be reliable where mothers gave the same answer on subsequent trials. The questionnaire is free of charge for anyone to use and has subsequently been the subject of several pilot projects and studies (listed in Box), and was used in a large study of over 2,000 infants who were presented to chiropractic offices in the UK. As such, the UKIQ has been found to be very user-friendly, both to parents and to practice, as well as scientifically valid and reliable.

List of studies done with the UKIQ to determine feasibility and relevant findings	
» Pilot project: Use in a chiropractic clinic (Schmid et al., 2016).	» Findings: In a University/College teaching clinic, mothers reported good results from the care of their infant and lowered depression scores.
» Is it useful in electronic format? (Hanson et al., 2018)	» This study showed that the form was usable in an electronic format in widespread offices.
» Which is preferred, electronic or paper? (Hiew et al., 2018)	» This study found that mothers preferred the electronic format.
» In 16 chiropractic practices, what are the results? (Miller et al., 2018)	» This study showed that the survey was useful in widespread offices and that mothers reported effectiveness of care, safety, and cost-effectiveness for their infant.

CHAPTER 4

What are the Outcomes of Infant Care in Chiropractic Practice? Adaptability of a Parent-Reported Outcome Measure to the Infant Population

Although millions of children are presented to chiropractors for care around the world each year, most commonly the infant, there are no previous large studies that show exactly who presents to the clinics, what their backgrounds and problems are, and what mothers report about treatment.

First, it must be said that mothers are excellent reporters of their child's issues and have, time and time again, been found to be accurate (Barr, Kramer, Boisjoly, McVey-White, & Pless, 2004; St. James-Roberts, 2008). Second, great effort was made in this study to avoid the "halo effect," a phenomenon where the patient rates a service higher than might be accurate to please the doctor or clinician. Consequently, the forms were completed in the absence of any healthcare representative to give the mother complete privacy so she could feel free to answer exactly as she felt.

It is also important to note that this was not a randomized-controlled trial (more on those later), which are considered high-quality trials and the only type that can state the actual effect of a treatment. The reason that blinded RCTs are high-level trials is that parents don't know whether their child was getting treated or not, and whether the babies are randomized to a treatment group or not. The problem with that type of trial is that it has no "external" validity, so that the results may not be relevant in the real world. Of course, such a trial can only compare the findings between 25 to 100 patients, so the numbers are small, and that is one reason that the findings, though helpful to determine the efficacy of treatment, are not the only way to determine results from treatment. They are often pooled into something called a systematic review, a high level of research. More will be discussed on that later, where they have been used to investigate infant crying.

External validity skyrockets in the Patient/Parent-Reported Outcomes-PROs type of study (the one we are describing right here). Thus, it seems very likely that the findings of this study should apply to other infants in similar situations, who are presented by their parents to a chiropractic clinic. In any event, the findings present real-world data (Katkade, Sanders, & Sou, 2018), which have been described as very credible in this current healthcare climate, and are likely much better to describe routine clinical outcomes than would a randomized, controlled trial. As such, the results do no more and no less than report what mothers stated about their baby's condition as they entered the clinic, and again at the end of an episode of treatment by the chiropractor. Each person can assess the data as they see fit, but it does most certainly reflect the real clinical world. All of the data were gathered prospectively, meaning at the time, so that no long-term recall was required. This improves the credibility of research findings.

There are tables and figures to help you look at the data. But I will also briefly describe it, clinician to clinician, so that you can get an overview of the findings.

Results of Maternal Report of Outcomes of Chiropractic Care for Her Infant

Just over half (55%, $n=1,092$) of the 2,001 infants parents brought to the clinics were boys, and this is standard in virtually all practices. Also common is the fact that about 2/3 of them had had one or more types of assisted births; that is, births that were not routine and natural but included medical interventions. Probably at least partly because of this, almost 60% of the infants were referred to chiropractors by other healthcare practitioners, most commonly midwives, general practice nurses, healthcare visitors, and occasionally by GPs or pediatricians. Babies often had multiple problems, but crying, feeding, and sleeping (particularly notable was difficulty lying on their back) were the most common complaints. Fortunately, mothers were able to check as many conditions as she had noted about their babies, so there were almost 4,400 complaints for 2,001 babies. This is not unusual, as it is well known that these problems often occur together (Hemmi et al., 2011). The average baby had just over two complaints. About 80% of babies were under 12 weeks of age. It has been noticed for years that the pediatric population attending chiropractic clinics is very young, with the under-1s having the largest representation (Hestbaek et al., 2009; Miller, 2010), and the most common age is just under 3 weeks (Jaskulski & Miller, 2018).

The profile of the infant who entered the office and the degree of their problems was interesting. But even more interesting was the mother's report of the degree of the problem(s) when they were released from the clinic (Box 3: Change of baseline ratings after treatment). The intake form asked mothers to report the level of pain, problems with sleep, crying, feeding, etc. along with their level of anxiety, depression, and quality of life for the baby and the family. The same questions were asked on the release form. It was remarkable that the mothers reported across-the-board improvements, with very robust percentages of improvement in the infant's condition, as well as the maternal level of anxiety and depression. All of the changes were tested for statistical significance and found to be significant to a very high degree, with a p-value < 0.0001. This can be interpreted that the likelihood that that much improvement could have occurred by chance was less than one chance out of a thousand. Thus, it was highly unlikely that even one baby in the entire population would have improved this much by pure chance.

Another way of looking at change was by a standard Global Index of Change (GIC). This is a common way of looking at a change in patients' condition over the time that they are in medical treatment. By this measure, over 82% were in the top two categories (which described a very significant level of change, called definite improvement, like a different baby, or completely better, and made a huge difference). We wanted to be very conservative in our interpretation, so we used only those top two categories, where there was no room for equivocal findings. However, if we look at the other categories, another 10% of mothers declared her baby to be moderately better or a little better (5%). Less than 3% of babies were unchanged or worse.

These positive changes or improvement in the baby's condition may have contributed to the very high ratings of satisfaction. Only 5% of mothers were not very satisfied or only somewhat satisfied.

The rest of the mothers rated their satisfaction very high, with over 70% in the very top rating (10 out of 10). Now, it is impossible to say what mothers mean by those ratings, and ideally, a qualitative study would follow to ask them what they meant when they ticked that box. Nevertheless, a real strength of the Patient-Reported Outcomes research is that it does allow the user of the healthcare service to have their say about their level of satisfaction, along with all of the rest of their opinions. Whether the satisfaction rates are high due to excellent clinical care, or something less important (to us), like short waits or easy parking, they are still very important in rating clinicians and finding differences between types of service. The mother's opinion should be valued and honored.

Perhaps an even better way to make comparisons, however, may be the question asked about cost-effectiveness. We asked a subset of about 500 mothers whether they found the care cost-effective. It is important here to keep in mind that this study took place in the UK, where chiropractic care bears a fee, compared to the National Health Service, which is free of charge. Still, 96% of mothers stated that the care was cost-effective. These opinions are now considered standard ways to compare types of service and to determine the value of the service for the patient. Thus, this is an excellent result, and the clinicians should be pleased that they provided value for money.

Of course, clinical improvement, satisfaction, and cost-effectiveness would have no value if the care had been found to be dangerous. Despite several calls and attempts to provide a prospective study of the safety of chiropractic care for infants, this was the first-known reported study with such a large sample. No adverse events were reported, and only rare side effects were reported. Side effects were whatever the mother thought was a side effect, so this was all about her perception, now considered an appropriate way to measure care.

The most common side effects were a mild increase in fussiness or irritability within the first 24 hours, greatly reduced to lower levels after that period, and better sleep after treatment. There were no adverse events (see box detailing, in the mother's words, any side effects from care).

As the first large-scale prospective study of safety of chiropractic care for infants, this is an important first step to other studies. It should be noted that until now, virtually all studies and all systematic reviews of safety of care have found that chiropractic care and manual therapy are safe procedures for infants and children (Todd, Carroll, Robinson, & Mitchell, 2015). However, these were all retrospective and systematic reviews. This is the first prospective study of a large sample of infants undergoing chiropractic care with good results and no adverse events (see Chapter 11, Safety, for details).

The average number of treatments was four over a two-week time span. The most common number of treatments was three. Because of the rapid change in the baby's condition, it can be said that the treatment was effective in a timespan that was much better than the "natural history" of the disorder. For example, infant excessive crying (also known as infant colic) has been said to resolve after 12 to 26 weeks of age. Since the average age of the presenting infant was 2 to 3 weeks of age, and the average number of weeks' treatment was two or less, the benefits of the treatment cannot easily be attributed to natural history or time alone. It can most likely be attributed to the care given to the baby.

There are figures and tables to give you further details in the mother's perceptions of her baby's care.

Baseline profile of infant patients presented to chiropractic clinics		
CHARACTERISTICS	**COUNT**	**PERCENT**
Gender (Total *n*=2,001)		
Male	1,092	55%
Female	909	45%
Type of Birth (Total *n*=1,808)		
Birth without Interventions	645	36%
Birth with Interventions	1,163	64%
Induced	415	22%
Ventouse	146	%8
Forceps	267	%15
Elective C-section	220	12%
Emergency C-section	290	%16
Assisted/Epidural	79	%4
Referral Patterns (Total *n*=1,689)		
Healthcare provider	989	58%
Friends and Family	485	29%
None or other	215	%13
Reason for Attendance (Total *n*=1,991)		
Crying	618	31%
Feeding	935	47%
Sleeping	495	25%
Uncomfortable when lying on back	536	27%
Unable to turn head equally to both sides	271	14%
Difficult birth	372	19%
Head shape	226	11%
Check up	448	23%
Reflux/Gas/Constipation	249	13%
Others	231	12%
Total	4,381*	
Average Number of Complaints	2.20	
Age in Weeks (Total *n*=1,842)		
12 weeks or below	1,583	86%
Above 12 weeks	259	14%

*Mothers could tick as many boxes as desired and could write in reason for attendance.

Mean change in maternal ratings from baseline to follow-up in infants presented to chiropractors for care				
CATEGORY RATED	RATING BEFORE TREATMENT	RATING AFTER TREATMENT	% CHANGE	P-VALUE
Feeding	3.93	1.26	-67.94%	p=0.0001
Sleeping	3.90	1.69	-56.67%	p=0.0001
Crying	3.67	1.48	-59.67%	p=0.0001
Supine sleep	4.21	1.61	-61.76%	p=0.0001
Infant pain	4.14	1.49	-64.01%	p=0.0001
Maternal anxiety	4.16	1.20	-71.15%	p=0.0001
Maternal depression	2.28	0.79	-63.35%	p=0.0001
Satisfaction with motherhood	2.75	1.16	-57.82%	p=0.0001
Cervical rotation	3.27	1.47	-55.05%	p=0.0001
Tummy time	3.52	4.64	31.82%	p=0.0001

Side effects listed by mothers after an
average of four chiropractic treatments for their infant

» Agitated just after treatment but much better the next day
» Slightly cranky on the night of treatment but much better the next day
» Cried one evening post-treatment for a couple of hours
» Unsettled at night more than normal
» Unsettled for one day only but back to content state
» Better sleep
» Upset that evening but difficult to tell if it's because of treatment
» Cried a little more one evening
» Unsettled after treatment for a few hours
» Lots of sleep, very nice side effect
» Slightly irritable after treatment for a few hours, then good sleep
» Tiredness after treatment
» After first jaw treatment, baby dribbled more but improved after second treatment
» A bit of fussiness
» Cranky after treatment at the beginning but now much more comfortable
» Was cranky after treatment and quite unsettled but only after the first two appointments
» Unsettled and difficult to console after treatment but rarely, and usually calm by the next day

CHAPTER 5

Inconsolable, Irritable Infants: The Highest Level of Evidence

This is probably where it all started. For many years (and I mean seven or more decades), distraught parents have brought screaming babies to chiropractors, demanding, "Do something!" And chiropractors did. The therapy seemed to work, and parents went off with a sleeping or drowsy, comfortable baby in their arms. What was that all about? Chiropractors have always been a practical sort of clinician who faced problems of pain with a biomechanical focus when other causes had been ruled out. After ruling out all pathology with history and examination, a trial of treatment was done. If it worked, the answer was simple; it was a biomechanical problem. The treatment was both safe and effective.

However, a curious Danish chiropractor in the 80s decided that the problem deserved further study (Klougart, Nilsson, & Jacobs, 1989). They did the first review of 316 cases and found that yes, chiropractic care seemed to be a solution for the excessively crying baby, which was called and still is, though erroneously, infant colic. The treatment worked, but why? Despite the proposed mechanisms that may successfully treat biomechanical constraint or musculoskeletal dysfunction in the child, there may be still myriad reasons as to why chiropractic treatment has been found effective for excessively crying babies. The following suggestions propose potential reasons. However, these should not be considered exhaustive or exclusive (see further details on the mechanics of care later).

1. Mechanical treatment redirects the musculoskeletal misalignment, and the baby becomes settled due to improved physical comfort.

2. The baby's autonomic nervous system is reset, calmed, or balanced, and the baby is emotionally comfortable.

3. Both of the above may work together.

There is continued search for therapies that work for infant colic. Pharmacology has demonstrated no benefits for the excessively crying baby in several double-blind studies (Lucasson, 2010). Therefore, the answer, so far, is not in taking drugs.

Manual skills, which individualize variable palpatory pressures, may uncover functional rather than pathological problems in the infant. The final common pathway of manual therapeutics performed on infants is one of release; joint release when immobility is observed and myofascial release when a muscle is hypertonic (tight or taut). When these are factors preventing normal biomechanical actions in children, they may feel relief with the release of the constraints of the tissue. Since birth trauma is the number-one risk for infant colic (Zwart, Velema-Goud, & Brand, 2005), it is most likely that this release of a restricted barrier in the tissue is the cause of relief for the baby.

What's in a Name? How Important Is Infant Colic?

First, it's important to clear up the name. Colic implies stomach pain (and huge problems in animals, such as horses, where it can be life-threatening). Wessel's team coined the term for the disorder in babies in 1950. Three symptoms diagnosed infant colic: crying more than three hours a day, more than three days a week, for more than three weeks. Note that this does not say anything about the digestive system. However, it was thought that "colicky" babies, which we will term *inconsolable, irritable infants (III)*, demonstrated some tension in the stomach (of course they did; they are crying) and probably expelled excess gas (they were increasing intrathecal tension with crying).

The name colic alone has brought endless issues for chiropractors who are treating musculoskeletal problems that are associated with irritability and **NOT** treating a digestive disorder. Is it time for an enlightened name change?

The reason to propose a name change is that the term "infant colic" presupposes that colic, or digestive colon disturbance, is implicated by definition (Dorland's Medical Dictionary, 2007, p. 389):

> Pertaining to the colon. Acute abdominal pain; characteristically, intermittent visceral pain with fluctuations corresponding to smooth muscle peristalsis.

This is one of the numerous myths about infant colic that need to be discarded (see Box on next page).

For some time, there has been considerable evidence accrued that the malady called infant colic has nothing to do with "colic" or irritation to the digestive system, showing no differences between colicky and non-colicky babies (Yalcin et al., 2010). In fact, X-rays showed there was less gas at the start of crying than at the end

(Illingsworth, 1985; Miller & Barr 1991). For many years, the condition was defined in terms of time of crying, rather than according to any specific symptoms (Wessel et al., 1954). The hallmark of infant colic is not merely excessive crying (which occurs in other conditions as well), but inconsolable crying concentrated at one time of the day, most commonly late afternoon, and evening to night time.

Historical myths of infant colic

» Infant colic is a syndrome reflecting upset in the digestive system, or colon.

» Infant colic is a benign syndrome with uneventful recovery by the end of 3 months.

» Infant colic is the end-range on a continuum of normal crying.

» Infant colic has no long-term effects on the parents or child.

» Infant colic is cow's milk protein intolerance or lactose intolerance.

» Infant colic is due to poor parenting.

» Infant colic only afflicts the firstborn and is related to inexperienced parenting.

» Boys and girls are afflicted similarly with infant colic and other crying syndromes.

Infant colic (IC), which has an evening peak, is known for its inconsolability and inconsolable nocturnal crying syndrome (INCS) might be a better term. Infant crying should only be called excessive when the reasons for the crying are unknown. For example, crying related to a painful urinary-tract infection should not be labeled as excessive crying. Once the reason is found and treated, the crying abates. The same is true for crying related to cow's milk protein intolerance (CMPI). Once understood and treated with the appropriate feed, then the crying subsides.

Excessive crying should only be termed so when the parent or clinician cannot understand the amount, extent, and intensity of crying, and that the amount of crying is dysfunctional for that baby. This underlines the fact that all infants should be examined for occult injury (Freedman, Al-Harthy, & Thull-Freedman, 2009), pathology, infection, or a problem that results in a context-specific cause of the crying before being termed an excessively crying or irritable infant with no known cause. Inconsolable nocturnal crying syndrome reasonably describes the concept of infant colic and excludes the misnomer of connection to the infant's colon. The name is important because it points out that the condition is not pathological and, therefore, approachable conservatively. No medical treatment has been found efficacious. Chiropractic care has shown good effect in treating the problem, with better effect than other treatments at this time. Chiropractors should take a back seat to no one in treating this condition. This is primarily because chiropractic treatment has been found to be safe, and therefore, could be an appropriate first-line option for parents to try. Still, it is very important to continue to research the causes and potential therapies for this problem.

Others have found a link between crying and pain, and called it a Pain Syndrome of Infancy (PSI). Gudmundson (2010) found a link between pain and excessive crying. Zwart et al. (2005) found that the most common risk for infant colic is a difficult birth. These both support the rationale for chiropractic treatment in that it treats a biomechanical discomfort, and when restored to normal, reduces crying time in the baby.

Inconsolable infant irritability has traditionally been termed infant colic. Although the terms have and continue to be used interchangeably, the term infant colic has been considered inappropriate because it does not describe the etiology of the crying and it has accrued many monikers, including simply crybabies, excessive crying of infancy, irritable-infant syndrome, unexplained infant crying, inconsolable crying of infancy, unsettled infant syndrome, or a pain syndrome of infancy. The condition has been described in the medical literature for over 70 years with the seminal work of Wessel (Wessel et al., 1954), calling it "3-months colic" because it was thought to remit spontaneously at 12 weeks of age. That timeline has since been revised upward with remission said to be anticipated at 4, 5, or 6 months of age and other authors stating that it does not remiss at all. The children's behavior simply changes as a wider repertoire of responses become available as they develop (Wolke et al., 2002). These children have been measured and described as continually unsettled at 7 to 8 months of age and to middle childhood (Sanson, Prior, & Oberklaid 1985; Wolke, Rizzo, & Woods, 2002).

Several research investigations (Becker, Holtmann, Laucht, & Schmidt, 2004; Hemmi, 2011; Rao, Brenner, Schistermann, Vik, & Mills, 2004; Savino et al., 2005; von Kries, Kalies, & Papousek, 2006; Wolke et al., 2002) note a long-term negative effect of infant colic from toddlerhood to school age. It has been implicated in maternal depression (Vik et al., 2009), severe stress in the family, difficulties in family communication, general dissatisfaction and sleeping disorders, as well as psychological disorders (Hall et al., 2011). Hence, the excessive, persistent crying of infant colic does not appear to be "benign and self-limiting," as some early authors (Wessel et al., 1954) have proposed.

Potential long-term sequelae are not the only reason for concern about the condition. Numerous authors (Carbaugh, 2004; Crouch,

2008; Minns, Jones, & Mok, 2008; Reijneveld, van der Wal, Brugman, Hira Sing, & Verloove-Vanhorick, 2004; Wirtz & Trent, 2008) have found a link between excessive crying and child abuse. Parents simply run out of ways to handle the baby who will not stop crying, no matter how voraciously they soothe. When investigated, parents who abused their child all gave the same reason; inability to stop the child's crying (Carbaugh, 2004).

Inconsolable crying of infancy requires attention. Despite this being the most common condition presented to clinicians in the first year of an infant's life, little respite has been afforded these children or their parents. As time has passed, another issue has become apparent. Fewer extended families are surrounding the infant to assist in care, and this as well can cause more difficulty to the family than would be the case if grandparents, aunts, and uncles were available to help hold and soothe the child.

Inconsolability of the child's cry is the hallmark of this condition, and it is often considered that the child is expressing pain or discomfort and has no other way to seek help. Hence, the inconsolable infant is an enigmatic problem with no known cause or cure. The rate of affliction is wide, ranging from 20% to 35% of infants (Hogdall, Vestermark, Birh, Plenov, & Toftager-Larson, 1991), and this may be attributable, in part, to the difficulty in defining the condition and its etiology. It is a leading cause of child abuse and is, therefore, of key importance to find a solution.

What is the Evidence for Chiropractic Manual Therapy for the Inconsolable, Irritable Infant (Infant Colic)?

The highest quality evidence in making treatment decisions comes from systematic reviews of randomized-controlled trials (RCTs) (Guyatt, 2016). RCTs are considered the gold standard of efficacy research and the power of the RCT comes from the randomization, as it is pure chance as to which patient goes into which arm of the trial. This procedure overcomes selection bias that can occur in studies where patients volunteer to participate in a study with a specific type of treatment. It controls for other biases, such as socioeconomic status of the family, inherent health risks or behaviors of the family, education, etc., as these factors are evenly distributed through the process of randomization. The RCT provides evidence that therapy works.

That said, RCTs are considered more reliable if the patients are blinded to the treatment condition. Otherwise, the mere promise of a new drug or treatment might have a placebo effect and the patient will get better due to hope, rather than the actual treatment. Ideally, the clinician is blinded as well, as doctors can be biased too. However, it is wellknown that some therapies are difficult to blind, such as surgery, acupuncture, and manipulation, because the doctor will know that they have performed the treatment.

The difficulty in blinding with manual therapy has been a problem for a long time, and this is the primary reason why most RCTs of infant colic have not been blinded. It is impossible to blind practitioners, as they will know whether or not they gave treatment. However, it is possible to blind the patient, or in this case, the parent. Infants are blinded to their treatment condition, as they do not possess the cognitive ability to make considerations about treatment vs. non-treatment (Haugen et al., 2011). It is at least theoretically possible that they might pick up "vibes" from the parent, but this does not cause a treatment effect not otherwise present. Therefore, the parent is the one who is blinded in these studies, although it is difficult because of a governing body mandatory requirement preventing separation of child and guardian (General Chiropractic Council, 2010) in the UK. We overcame that rule in our UK study in a novel way, which I will describe later.

Several studies testing manual treatment for infant colic have shown a positive result (Browning & Miller, 2008; Hayden & Mullinger, 2006; Karpelowsky, 2004; Koonin, Karppelowsky, Yelverton, & Rubens, 2005; Mercer & Nook, 1999; Miller, 2012; Wiberg, Nordsteen, & Nilsson, 1999). One study did not (Olafsdottir, Forshei, Fuge, & Markestad, 2001). Olafsdottir's study is one of the trials that attempted parental blinding, and whether true or not, this has been considered to be the reason for the difference in results. However, there were many other significant differences in their trial, and therefore, Cochrane reviewed it as an "outlier," done differently than the other trials. The main differences in this trial were, among others:

1. All of the babies had severe-level crying and had been referred from other clinicians who had previously treated the child. Therefore, these were not routine cases of infant colic but were most likely sensory-disordered children, or what we have called "IFCIDS": Irritable Feeding Crying Infants with Disordered Sleep. In other words, these were babies on the far spectrum of inconsolable infants, not the routine cases that come into a chiropractic office on a daily basis. In our 2012 study, we found that these babies only modestly improve (Miller & Newell, 2012).

2. The cervical spine was not examined or treated by the clinician.

3. There was only one treating clinician.

4. The treating clinician once claimed that if he had set out to prove that chiropractic care did not help infants, he was in a position to do that. (This can be considered hearsay, though he did say it to me, and I am NOT claiming that that is what he set out to do, that is what the study did.)

5. There was a limit of three treatments for each child, instead of a treatment protocol that matched each case. In our study of IFCIDS, we found that they needed much more treatment than infant colic and even then, the results were not as consistent (Miller & Newell, 2012).

6. The babies who were not treated were held and rubbed through the spine to still them and calm them. In other studies, untreated babies were untouched. It is considered best not to treat infants in the control group at all, particularly when it is known that touch may ease pain (Honda et al., 2013).

7. The result of this trial is that all of the babies cried less, the treatment group less than the control group, but not to a statistically significant degree.

8. The trial did not use the gold-standard crying diary, although there was some report that they did.

Therefore, it was necessary to do another blinded trial to continue to test the power of blinding in this type of care. Some have said that blinding of the parent is not essential because all parents, in their fatigue and confusion over the crying child, may not know if their child is treated or not. In fact, in our experience, after a treatment (probably due to comfortable care, light touch, and low-force methods), parents sometimes ask, "did you actually do anything?" Only after they see the change in their child's behavior are they reassured that there was a treatment.

Hence, our RCT was conceived with the goal of overcoming weaknesses from the other trials. It was not possible to overcome some specific weaknesses of the Olafsdottir trial because their trial did not divulge sufficient detail to understand the actual procedures of the study. We have had to glean these through questions and comments heard at seminars.

Lack of transparency in scientific trials creates problems for others who wish to overcome specific sources of bias. However, bias is, perhaps, inevitable, no matter how well-designed the study. Our subsequent study aimed to reduce as much bias as possible in assessing the therapeutic benefit of chiropractic treatment for the infant patient suffering from excessive crying.

The trial we designed did undertake blinding. Because the General Chiropractic Council in the UK does not allow parents to be separated from the underage child during treatment, the treatment rooms contained an opaque floor-to-ceiling screen that the parents could not see around. The parents were in the same room for legal reasons but could not view the treatment to satisfy the protocol of the trial. For further protection, the parents were given paperwork to concentrate on during the treatment (and they often stared into their telephone). All treating and non-treating clinicians were given a script so that all parents heard vocal dialog that suggested that the baby had a treatment. The non-treating clinicians also had paperwork assignments to assure that they would keep their hands off the child. There was also an observing clinician in the room.

The outcomes of the trial were that infants who were treated cried significantly less than those who were not treated, whether the parents were blinded or not. It can be argued that there is added strength to the result when the method changes (blinding versus non-blinding) and the results are the same. Thus, it may be appropriate that other trials, which were not blinded, should be re-interpreted in light of new information from this trial. Blinding of the parent does not appear to be essential.

The Miller-UK trial had key findings:

1. Excessively crying infants who are treated with chiropractic manual therapy improve to a statistically significant degree over those who are not treated.

2. Reduced crying occurred whether the parents were blinded or not. Therefore, blinding of the parents is not necessary to obtain good results for the baby and to show that the therapy is effective.

3. Babies also slept more and better after the treatment. This was not a focused outcome of our study, so we did not report it as such. However, Cochrane reviewers studied sleep as well and stated that babies treated with manual therapy do achieve better sleep patterns, to a statistically significant degree (Dobson et al., 2012).

As in other trials, the response from the baby occurred very quickly, within 10 days of treatment. The initial response occurred very early, within the first six days of therapy and after 1.1 treatments. This was a major learning event from the trial (and a drawback as well). We learned that parents whose baby does not get better straight away, within the first six days, will not stay for more treatment, but will seek other types of care. From this, we learned that the problem is considered so severe that it needs attention, and that it works and works immediately. We learned that babies start to get better quickly, after just 1.1 treatments. This reassured the parents of babies who were treated to continue with the treatment.

Our study was the strongest trial so far of chiropractic care for crying babies. There were several strengths that subsequent studies should consider:

1. Other causes of excessive infant crying were ruled out before entering the trial. This was the first trial to treat only "infant colic" and not other conditions, which may appear to be the classic inconsolable-infant condition but must be differentially diagnosed.

2. The non-treatment (control) group was not touched by the clinicians. This was a major strength in that clinicians may, even inadvertently, treat or intend to treat simply because the drive to help and heal is so strong. We could not be sure that clinicians would refrain from any intention to treat, so we insisted on total abstinence in the protocol.

3. Therefore, this was a test of the actual manual treatment for the child, not of good intentions, or of the reassurance that a parent may feel by bringing their child to a modern office with a good reputation, where they pay for treatment and expect good results. The aspects of the Halo effect or expectations were removed because:

    a. there was no payment for the treatment,

    b. the parent did not know whether the child was treated or not,

   c. the parent could see in the crying diaries with immediate effect whether the treatment actually helped or not, and

   d. the crying diary, which is considered the gold standard to determine the treatment effect or not, was used in this trial.

5. Side effects of care were gathered prospectively, and there were no adverse events. Better sleep was the chief side effect of care. They also showed improved sleep in the diaries.

This trial was included in a Cochrane Systematic Review (Dobson et al., 2012) of manual therapy for infant colic and given an honorable mention. A systematic review is considered the highest level of evidence. There have been several reviews of colic trials, but this one was done at the highest level and remains the most respected. That said, there was a major drawback. Cochrane did not include the unblinded treatment arm in their meta-analysis. This gave the trial half as much power and therefore, the actual results from the manual treatment for the babies was much better than used in the Cochrane meta-analysis. If all treated babies had been used in the final analysis, the outcome would likely have reached an even more significant outcome. More trials are still required.

Their findings concur that yes, manual therapy is effective for colicky babies and that they will cry one hour and 12 minutes less per day after the treatment. This can be viewed in something called a Forest Plot (see below).

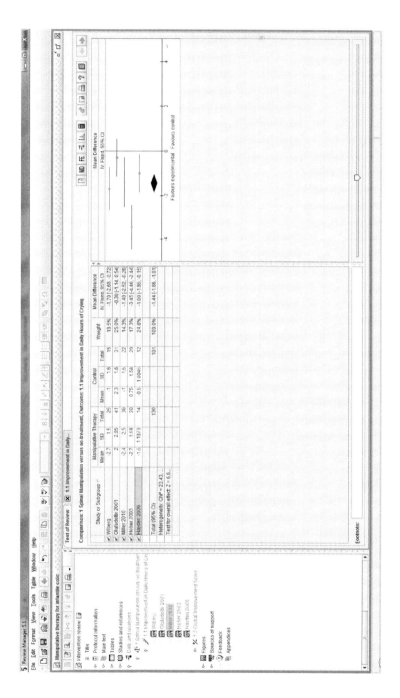

The Forrest Plot shows that those on the left of the midline had found benefit from the treatment. These are the babies that had manual therapy. The one trial that crossed the midline (point of no effect) is the Norwegian study, where all babies improved, but not significantly.

My thought is that the Norwegian study did not, in fact, study colic babies, but IFCIDS (see Miller & Newell, 2012 for the common causes of crying babies). The babies in their trial had all been previously treated and referred in. This is the same as the group of IFCIDS in the Miller study. It is plausible that they were not treating actual colicky babies, which they had set out to study. Their findings were the same as the 2012 Miller and Newell study, where IFCIDS did get better, but to a less significant degree than the colicky babies.

Until or unless there is conclusive evidence, there is sufficient evidence that chiropractic care works for the crying baby to support the treatment and to suggest its use for the inconsolable infant. Because it is a safe treatment (see the evidence about safety), it is an appropriate way forward. Even if it does not help every baby, it will not hurt, according to the evidence and therefore, a therapeutic trial is a good way forward that might help parents' suffering a great deal. Other studies show that mothers of crying babies report less anxiety and depression when their infant is treated in a chiropractic clinic (Marrilier, Lima, Donovan, Taylor, & Miller, 2014; Schmid, Hetlevik, & Miller 2016). This is a significant benefit and would stand alone, even if babies did not cry less with care (which, of course, studies show that they do).

CHAPTER 6

Are There Long-Term Problems With Inconsolable Infants?

W hat if babies with excessive crying problems are not treated? Some, no doubt, grow out if it, or express their issues more acceptably. But others may turn to different types of more age-appropriate dysfunctional behaviors to manage their discomfort.

Several studies demonstrate negative long-term sequelae in older children who suffered from infant colic as a baby (Becker et al. 2004; Hemmi et al., 2011; Papousek & von Hofacker, 1998; Rautava, Lehtonen, Helenius, & Sillanpaa, 1995; Rao, Brenner, Schisterman, Vik, & Mills, 2004; von Kries et al., 2006; Wolke et al., 2002). These risks start almost immediately in the early weeks of life, when not only are infants with colic at increased risk of being taken off breastfeeding in the hopes that formula-feeding will stop the crying, but they are often put on solids very early, without benefit and with potential harm (Howard, Lanphear, Lanphear, Eberly, & Lawrence, 2006). This can cause other health problems associated with feeding other than the gold standard of breastfeeding (see Chapter 8). Excessive crying is also the most common cause of infant abuse (Carbaugh, 2004).

It is no longer accepted that infant colic is transient and harmless. Rather, it increases the risk of behavioral problems in childhood (Hemmi et al., 2011). Children who have suffered from colic appear to have decreased capacity for self-regulatory behavior for months or even years after the colicky episode. For example, Rautava et al. (1995) found significant differences in family functioning in post-colic toddlers versus children who did not have colic as infants.

Although multiple studies show long-term behavioral problems in children who suffered from colic in infancy, what has not been investigated is whether successful treatment has any effect on the long-term ramifications. We did such a study in the UK twice, partly because we did not believe the results the first time since they were so clear-cut that early treatment made a long-term difference. The results, in effect, were too good to be true. Within a student project, questionnaires were sent to 129 families three years after their infant had been treated for colic in a chiropractic teaching clinic. Results indicated that those who had been treated successfully (by parent report) had significantly fewer temper tantrums and sleep disturbances compared to findings reported in the research literature (Hagh, 2005). The study was not submitted for publication because it did not include a control group for comparison of children who had had no treatment and we felt that the bias might, therefore, be too great.

With the thought that there must be too much bias in the study that attributed long-term benefits for early treatment of inconsolable infants, we did a second study. We added a control group to look at the differences. *Journal Manipulative and Physiological Therapeutics* published this study in 2009, authored by Miller and Phillips. The methodology is described below.

Approximately 200 children, all between 2 and 3 years of age, were surveyed with half having had successful chiropractic treatment for excessive crying during early infancy, and half having had colic as a baby with no effective treatment. The results showed that children treated by chiropractors displayed significantly less disruptive behavior than the control group at 2 to 3 years of age. These children fed better, slept better, and had fewer temper tantrums than the untreated groups. This was in exact agreement with the earlier research.

Although a comparative-cohort study is not as strong as the RCT, it was the only type of study that could answer the question of whether there were long-term benefits of chiropractic care for children. As such, this is the most accessed article in the series of publications used in this research. The reason for this is, most likely, because other studies show that inconsolable, irritable infants have significantly difficult behavior traits as toddlers. What is unique about this study is that these babies, when treated successfully by chiropractors, do not display those difficult behaviors in toddlerhood.

Even at this point, it remains only the second and most methodologically sound study of its kind. Moreover, both studies showed the same trends. Research suggests that manual therapy is a credible treatment for babies with painful problems. But we must further ask, what about babies who are not suffering from actual colic? Even then, how does it work?

CHAPTER 7

How to Differentially Diagnose Inconsolable, Irritable Infants

P arents ask, "Why is my baby crying incessantly? Why does he not stop despite my every effort at soothing him? What is the cause of the crying? Is he in great pain? Does he sleep too little because he cries all of the time? How much crying is too much crying?"

The inconsolable infant is one of the great enigmas in life. It has incited numerous "solutions," including the "cry it out" method, meaning leaving the baby on his own to cry until he stops. My theory is that he finally stops out of exhaustion and realizes that no one cares enough to listen to him, and there is no point in carrying on (learned helplessness). Although there is no evidence that these babies turn into axe murderers, loners, or the psychologically disabled, it seems plausible that there are more baby-friendly ways to deal with inconsolable infant crying. There is evidence that if they are treated successfully (to cry normally; we are NOT trying to stop crying), they have fewer problems in toddlerhood (Miller & Phillips, 2009).

Some professionals advocate leaving babies alone to "cry it out," no matter how long it takes to stop, and they do sometimes suggest it to harried parents. I find that method repulsive. The approach that I prefer (and this is purely from a clinical point of view, when an irritable baby is presented to my office) is to diagnose the cause of the problem and treat it to determine whether this alleviates the issue. If it does, the cause was found, and the problem is solved. If it does not, further investigation or referral is required. This leads to the need to correctly diagnose the baby.

Clinicians everywhere have been faced with the enigmatic crying baby, who seems quite healthy on the surface, but spends more than two, or even more than three, hours a day, most days, in abject, unstoppable crying, even screaming. The reason that this baby is thought to be healthy is that crying increases the use of oxygen by at least 10%, and some robust health is required for the ability to sustain the crying. As a clinician, I always say that I much prefer a severely crying baby to one who does not (because he cannot) cry at all. Inability to activate a boisterous cry is more likely to be part of a pathological problem, with a serious cause that requires immediate medical attention.

Some research has been done to differentially diagnose crying babies. Diagnosing the crying baby has presented clinicians with a conundrum for decades (Douglas & Hill, 2011). Although it is clear that very few excessively crying infants have a life-threatening illness (Freedman et al., 2009), further clarity as to etiology of the crying is notably lacking. We decided to do two studies to further diagnosis in our clinic. Defining characteristics, if not exact etiology, would be the first step toward subgrouping infants afflicted with the condition. Therefore, the rationale for our first diagnostic study was to determine which characteristics could reliably be associated with infant colic.

This first effort toward subgrouping was a novel study that used all characteristics previously associated in the research literature with infant colic. We surveyed over 1,000 parents who presented babies with infant crying and asked them to tick which characteristics were representative of their child (Kvitvaer, Miller, & Newell, 2010). By applying logistic regression, the risks for the condition could be suggested. A nomogram, a predictive tool often used in healthcare (Gorlia et al., 2008), was used to demonstrate the association between the clusters of features elicited. This was the first time that an attempt was made, using a large sample, to sequester the specific features that most correlate with the affliction. An important feature of this work is that it moved the clinical science beyond a diagnosis based on time of crying, three hours a day, which is much less specific and thus, less utilitarian. The strengths of this study were the maternal perceptions of the condition and the relatively small number of infants who presented without the condition (all of which were detailed within the study itself). These findings were used, in a preliminary way, to begin the important process of subgrouping the excessively crying infant.

The second and more clinically useful study was the *a priori* (meaning "in advance") subgrouping of excessively crying infants in categories based on previous research and clinical continuity. These groups could then be tested by collecting the data on success or failure of the chiropractic care for the condition of presentation. This was an excellent test of the theories.

There is an evidence base for doing this type of research. There are two ways to determine subgroups. The first is to identify the group with baseline characteristics before the start of a study. The second is to isolate the subgroups based upon unique or differing reactions to the treatment. The first might be considered less biased, and hence, *a priori* subgrouping was used in this study. Also, post-analysis subgrouping was used to inform unique aspects of each cluster. However, the post-analysis was not unplanned (which, according to Scott and Campbell in 1998, has more likelihood of resulting in selection bias). Instead, the statistical analyses were pre-planned, based on biological plausibility, and no overall statements of treatment effect were made. In short, we worked to create the least biased study possible.

Treatment efficacy could not be ascertained from this type of study because of the lack of randomization. Moreover, the study aimed to provide evidence for subgrouping, rather than prove therapeutic effectiveness, although it might give guidance in that direction.

Despite *a priori* decisions, it should be noted that it is also possible to uncover a subgroup effect not recognized before the start of the study. Certainly, in this study, it was not anticipated that there might be a subgroup with a better response to chiropractic therapy than infant colic, since past research has indicated good effectiveness of manual therapy for that condition. The subgroup irritable infants of musculoskeletal origin (IISMO; Chapter 9) showed some indications that manual treatment had a better effect than with infant colic.

This is, at this moment, considered a significant trend. The effect was found in post-analysis and contributed to the discussion of the mechanism of action or biological plausibility, in that some conditions are so clearly musculoskeletal in origin, it cannot be denied (IISMO). The link of infant colic to biomechanical fault is also a current concept (Wiberg & Wiberg, 2010). This discovery raises the possibility that clinical trials of infant colic may have included infants with other diagnoses, who should have been excluded. This study should be helpful to other studies in determining their inclusion and exclusion criteria for randomized trials.

Another aspect of this study was the attempt to capture the parent's stress level as a parameter of distress within the mother/infant dyad and as a clinical outcome measure. The patient's viewpoint and self-report (Fischer et al., 1999) have been found to be useful for some time in medical care, and prospective reports are sensitive to show change. It was the end of treatment change (reported prospectively, at the time), which was assessed in our subgrouping trial. Hirji and Fagerland in 2009 outlined the importance of outcome-based subgroup analysis, which has been used in our trial.

Other authors (Douglas & Hill, 2011) suggested that parents complain of lack of accessibility to any type of helpful healthcare, along with inconsistency of advice when they do access clinical help, and this is because clinicians do not understand the parameters of the condition, nor do they always refer to other healthcare professionals if they do not know how to resolve the problem. They point out that help should be sought early, before the behavior problems become entrenched in the child and stress builds within the family unit. It stands to reason that the earlier the problem is identified, the sooner it can be dealt with appropriately.

Our research aimed to demonstrate specific features of the excessively crying baby that could be recognized early. Another main objective was to facilitate pragmatic subgrouping of inconsolable, irritable infants. Subgrouping would facilitate a direct focus on the specific condition, rather than the amorphous group defined by crying time that constitutes the most commonly used diagnostic feature today. Crying time alone is not helpful, as there may be profoundly different causes of the crying. The crying is merely the final common pathway.

How to Subgroup Excessively Crying Babies

I suggest some obvious categories for the excessively crying baby:

1. **Pathology:** This could be anything causing pain to the baby. The most likely cause might be urinary tract infection. Pathology affects less than 5% of babies (Freedman et al., 2005), but pathology of any kind must be the first rule out for the clinician when presented with a crying baby. These babies will most commonly have a recent onset of crying. Crying is severe and relentless, often high-pitched, suggesting serious pain, and may be accompanied by a high temperature, high respiratory rate and heart rate, and/or more sleep, grogginess, or difficulty waking. This requires immediate referral for medical care. This is a very small percentage of infants attending a chiropractic clinic. My experience is <1%. Still, it is exceedingly important not to miss them and to refer them to appropriate care. Vital signs will be the first step in ruling out pathology.

2. **Cow's-milk protein intolerance (CMPI):** This may be pain induced by discomfort secondary to trying to digest the large proteins in cow's milk. Although this is more likely in artificially-fed babies than breastfed babies, it can also occur in breastfed babies if the mother ingests significant amounts of milk. The test is to remove the dairy products and see if the baby recovers. It can take up to a week to get the dairy completely out of the baby's system, but the behavior will change as soon as the offending substance is gone. The baby may show signs of allergy, reddening of the skin, high respiratory rate and noisy respiration, and either copious diarrhea or

constipation-type diapers. The only treatment is to remove the offensive substance, either through the removal of dairy from the mother's diet or to change the baby's formula to a hydrolyzed (90% reduction in large proteins) or amino-acid formula.

3. **The severity of the baby's allergy will determine which therapy is most workable:** Either way, this is a specific problem with a specific cause, which has nothing to do with infant colic. I estimate that these babies account for 5% to 10% of babies attending a chiropractic office and they can be easily differentially diagnosed and treated (Miller & Weber-Hellstenius, 2013).

4. **Irritable Infant Syndrome of Musculoskeletal Origin:** The hallmark of this pure MSK condition is usually a difficult birth, a twin, or history of intra-uterine constraint. These babies are most likely to cry when they cannot reach an antalgic posture of comfort. They may have tactile defensiveness (sensitive to touch), restless sleep (often unable to rest easily in a supine position), or difficulty to rest in a car seat. These babies do very well with chiropractic care because it is a manual therapy for musculoskeletal conditions and this is a pure musculoskeletal condition (Miller & Newell, 2012). This is a very common presentation to a chiropractic office, perhaps about 30% to 50% of the inconsolable irritable infants. Another variation of MSK problems in infancy is called KISS syndrome, as defined by Heiner Bierderman.

5. **Inefficient Feeding Crying Infant with Disordered Sleep (IFCIDS):** These are babies 1 to 6 months of age or even older, with many episodes of high-intensity crying, painful looks, body unrest, arching posture (not related to reflux), which can occur at any time of the day or night. The baby may awaken with intense crying. Both feeding and sleeping are affected. There is a male predominance of 60:40. This is not easily treated (Miller & Newell, 2012), and may be the crying condition that does not remit and continues through to toddlerhood and school age. This may be or become a sensory disturbance in the child. I estimate that this issue presents in about 15% to 20% of inconsolable infants in the chiropractic office. In our office, it was 16% of the inconsolable infants.

6. **Infant Colic:** Onset is most common between 2 to 10 days, certainly within the first two weeks of life. Loud, disturbing, relentless crying occurs often in late afternoon/evening. The abdomen is tense, and the arms and legs flail. Crying can continue unabated, whether picked up and soothed, or not. The baby generally sleeps well, eats well, and grows well. Research has shown in several randomized trials that this is treatable with chiropractic care and manual therapy. I estimate that this condition may be diagnosable in about 30% to 50% of inconsolable irritable infants entering a chiropractor's office.

The first two conditions may present to chiropractors but are not treatable with manual therapy. The last three conditions are treatable with manipulation. In our study, we found that so-called colic required the fewest number of treatments (3 to 4), followed by IISMO (6.6), and IFCIDS (7 or more). The results were an almost total resolution for IISMO, excellent recovery for colic, and only some improvement with IFCIDS. All of this supports the conclusion by Hughes and Bolton (2000) that there is good evidence that taking a crying baby to a chiropractor will result in less crying. This study suggests that when the problem is MSK in origin, then the baby improves with MSK treatment. What could be more logical? This makes clinical sense. That is why a condition that is pure MSK (IISMO or KISS) responds very well to manual therapy. Infant colic also responds very well, but slightly less than IISMO. This is evidence, of sorts, that the early onset crying of so-called infant colic is caused by biomechanical imbalances stemming from a difficult birth, not from a digestive disorder. Because of the difficulty of differential diagnosis, it is most likely that some of these cases in colic trials were misdiagnosed and were not, in fact, true colic babies. This will always be the case because of the inherent difficulty of differential diagnosis.

IFCIDS are most likely children with a primary sensory disorder, who find it difficult to settle. However, all of the incessant crying for those many weeks may have induced a musculoskeletal irritant or two as well. When these are treated, the baby may get slightly better, but that is not the complete answer. I have previously suggested that many of the children in the Norwegian trial were, in fact, IFCIDS and not infant colic. I suggest that chiropractors faced with this condition consult a book by Faure and Richardson (2008) for help to understand and to diagnose this child.

In our clinical trials, parents felt better, and rated their anxiety as lowered, with care (Marriller et al., 2015; Miller & Newell, 2012; Schmid et al., 2016). It is plausible that changes in parents' stress either precedes or follows decreases in crying. Whether it is the chicken or the egg, it is a good outcome. However, this did not occur to any great degree with the **IFCIDS** group, so it is more likely that parents' decreased stress is the result of a baby who cries less, rather than just an appearance at the clinic. If that were the case, the parent's stress level would reduce at presentation at any clinic for care, and this has never been shown to happen. In fact, it may be that stress levels in parents rise after seeking care and no help was given.

As we stated in the article, there is some plausibility to the findings of this study (Miller & Newell, 2012). Colic babies cry a great deal, particularly at the time of the day when biorhythms are lowest (end of the day) but do eat well, sleep well, and grow. True to their reputation, they were least consolable at the start. When they were treated successfully, they stopped the incessant crying and changed to what is considered a normal amount of crying for a baby (around 2 hours or less, with most, if not all, of it consolable). IISMO babies cried a great deal, but were consolable when held or positioned in the "correct" way for comfort, but did not sleep particularly well if they were required to sleep supine (important for the Back-To-Sleep program to prevent **SIDS**). There was no problem with growth. In fact, these children were, if anything, large for their age and presented older than the colic babies. Their **MSK** problems could have stemmed from a difficult birth as a large baby, or they may have been overfed in an attempt to stop the crying. IFCIDS presented slightly older as well. IFCIDS cried the most, slept the least, and also reported problems with feeding. These babies were usually on the lowest levels of the growth charts. There are no obese **IFCIDS**, at least in infancy. However, in an attempt to console them, babies could be overfed. It must also be kept in mind that babies could have more than one problem, such as both biomechanical colic and **CMPI**.

Improvement in sleeping is a common finding in babies who are treated with manual therapy. Parents reported significant improvements in sleep in all of our studies, in a randomized comparison study of 43 infants treated for excess crying (Browning & Miller, 2005). The Cochrane (2012) review unequivocally stated that infants who are treated with manual therapy sleep better.

This subgrouping study went some way to the differential diagnosis of the crying baby. Not every inconsolable infant should be diagnosed with infant colic; their characteristics need to be closely discerned to observe for other etiologies of crying. The chiropractor is well-placed to differentially diagnose, triage, and treat these babies with a biomechanical component of the discomfort.

CHAPTER 8

Babies
Who Cannot
Feed

The benefits of breastfeeding are well-known. It is the perfect food for babies, designed especially for their needs and contains all of the water and specific nutrients required in a bioavailable package. Artificial-formula companies spend millions trying to mimic breastmilk, without great success. Breastfed babies, statistically speaking (always leaving space for individual differences), are healthier and maintain their weight more easily (less childhood obesity) than artificially-fed babies. This is not the least of which because mother's milk contains the immunological properties required by the infant to maintain health. It is no wonder that mothers can feel quite distraught when they cannot breastfeed their baby.

When mothers cannot breastfeed, they tend to take all of the blame and say that it is their problem. Mothers' feelings have been quite difficult to document because excellent records are not often kept on the breastfeeding dyad. It is a very personal issue. There is a high uptake of breastfeeding at birth (about 88%), but a quick change to formula-feeding by 3 weeks of age. Babies who were born with one or more interventions were more likely to switch to formula-feeding (Homdrum & Miller, 2015). More than half of those who stopped breastfeeding reported biomechanical problems (Herzaft-LeRoy, Xhignesse, & Gaboury, 2018).

After birth, babies generally need to demonstrate that they are able to feed in the hospital before leaving for home. However, abilities to feed may fall off as soon as babies are released and then parents present their newborn to a variety of clinicians, including GPs, health visitors, midwives, lactation consultants, and then they are often referred to chiropractors, particularly if a biomechanical fault is suspected. Many clinicians may not feel confident about the diagnosis or treatment of a musculoskeletal fault that occurred from birth, that is irritating the feeding process. There is a very short time when an intervention can be effective because of early cessation, and turn to the bottle, usually at or before 3 weeks of age.

It is difficult to attain definitive evidence about the help that chiropractors can offer to the breastfeeding dyad. This is because it is impossible to perform a randomized-controlled trial in breastfeeding, simply because it would be unethical to deprive infants of any care that could help. Further, there is too much evidence, at this point, that biomechanical type of care does work to allow any child into a non-treatment category. The box on the next page shows a list of research that has been done showing some benefit of chiropractic care for infant-feeding problems. The largest of these studies was done in our clinic, and I will give the results below.

Published studies that evidenced success in breastfeeding for babies treated with chiropractic care
Tow & Vallone, 2009
Miller et al., 2009
Arcadi, 1993
Bernard et al., 2012
Cuhel & Powell, 1997
Fry, 2014
Hewitt, 1999
Holleman & Knaap, 2011
Holtrop, 2000
Hubbard, 2014
Sheader, 1999
Stewart, 2012
Vallone, 2004
Willis, 2011
Miller et al., 2009
Miller et al., 2016
Miller et al., 2018

In 2009, a cohort of infants was studied, who were all referred to the chiropractic clinic from other healthcare professionals. That referral confirmed that the infants presented all had moderate-to-severe problems with breastfeeding, which were unresolvable with the previous healthcare treatment. The mean age of infants by the time they reached the chiropractor was 3.2 weeks (with a range of 2 days to 12 weeks). The problems that were presented and treated were as follows:

» Altered tongue action resulting in an ineffective latch, but not due to tongue-tie

» Decreased mandible excursion

» Inability to tilt head into extension to allow wide-mouth opening

» Displaced hyoid preventing balanced tongue activity

» Aberrant cervical range of motion and/or posterior joint restrictions affecting infant posture and position

» Hypo or hypertonic orbicularis oris masseter, digastric muscles causing an imbalance in muscle torque

» Temporomandibular joint laxity or imbalance

» Mechanical changes in neural functions relative to cranial or cervical distortion

Although 41% of those attending had recorded an assisted birth, there were approximately 3 to 4 times as many ventouse and forceps extractions in these babies compared to the local hospital averages. Many of these infants had been seen by up to five healthcare practitioners, so it is very likely that other problems that were not biomechanical in origin had been ruled out. Histories of these babies included common injuries from birth, which are considered routine:

» Abrasions and blisters on face, scalp, buttocks, or genitals (breech) due to forceps; hematomas due to ventouse

» Punctures from scalp electrodes or incisions for fetal blood samples

» Petechiae due to prolonged labor, on head, neck, conjunctiva, or where cord wrapped around neck; asymmetries due to positioning

» Clavicle and skull fractures

When these types of superficial injuries are present, it must be suspected that there may be underlying injuries as well, not so easily diagnosed, but that may be causing the problems with feeding. In this case, biomechanical problems were found in the babies presented.

There was only one outcome measure, and that was exclusive breastfeeding. Therefore, any baby who improved to partial breastfeeding was not counted in the final positive results. This may have been unfair to some mothers, who did not choose total breastfeeding and may have chosen to combination feed. Also, a few of the babies were very old before being referred, and consequently, it may have been difficult to return to total breastfeeding.

In all, 78% of the babies were able to exclusively breastfeed at the end of treatment. The average number of treatments was four, and the most common number was three over a 10-day time frame. This is a relatively small study showing good results from co-treatment (chiropractic care after other types of healthcare) of infants with breastfeeding problems. In the UK, at 6 weeks, only 23% of infants are getting any breastmilk. In comparison, this was most likely a highly motivated group of mothers who wanted to sustain breastfeeding enough to keep going until they found someone who could help. Multiple practitioners are often consulted, and it can take this to enable successful breastfeeding. In my opinion, the most important factor for success is the motivated mother.

In an allied interdisciplinary feeding clinic in this same institution, another study was conducted and published in 2016, showing benefits for babies consulting a team of midwives and chiropractors. This study was published in an open access journal, and therefore, content can be reproduced. Here is the abstract from that study:

This service evaluation investigated an interdisciplinary allied professional health care strategy to address the problem of suboptimal breastfeeding. A clinic of midwives and chiropractors was developed in a university-affiliated clinic in the United Kingdom to care for suboptimal feeding through a multidisciplinary approach. No studies have previously investigated the effect of such an approach. The aim was to assess any impact to the breastfeeding dyad and maternal satisfaction after attending the multidisciplinary clinic through a service evaluation. Eighty-five initial questionnaires were completed and 72 (85%) follow-up questionnaires were returned. On follow-up, 93% of mothers reported an improvement in feeding as well as satisfaction with the care provided. Prior to treatment, 26% of the infants were exclusively breastfed. At the follow-up survey, 86% of mothers reported exclusive breastfeeding. The relative-risk ratio for exclusive breastfeeding after attending the multidisciplinary clinic was 3.6 (95% confidence interval 2.4-5.4) (Miller et al., 2016).

The relative-risk ratio means that babies attending the clinic were from 2.4 to 5.4 times as likely to breastfeed successfully after attending the clinic.

Further, the mothers who attended this clinic reported very high satisfaction rates with the interventions of both midwifery and chiropractic care. It is likely that this was a very highly motivated population who sought out this type of innovative clinic and this could account for the success rate, along with the treatments. We anticipate that as time goes by, the cases seen in chiropractic clinics become more and more complex as mothers seek wider and wider care. Chiropractors need to update their knowledge regularly in taking care of the breastfeeding dyad, just as other health professionals, most notably IBCLCs (International Board Certified Lactation Consultants) who often work side by side with manual therapists (Tow & Vallone, 2009). IBCLCs should be the first contact for babies with difficulty breastfeeding.

Many chiropractors have found their niche in understanding and treating the baby with breastfeeding dysfunction. Others may not know where to start. It is important to note that early cessation of breastfeeding is often associated with a difficult or assisted birth (Hall et al., 2002; Smith, 2007) and understanding the birth can help the doctor understand the biomechanical fault.

If there is a history of physiologic birth injury in the infant or birth intervention, the birth may be implicated in the difficulty to breastfeed. Breastfeeding is very important to the health of the newborn, as well as the mother.

Breastfeeding reduces the risks of:

- » Otitis media

- » Atopic dermatitis

- » Gastroenteritis

- » Respiratory Tract Infection

- » Asthma

- » SIDS

- » Leukemia

- » Diabetes

- » Rheumatoid Arthritis

- » Obesity

And improves:

- » Cognitive function (IQ)

- » Vascular function

- » Normal growth

- » Attachment/bonding

(Ip, Chung, Raman, et al., 2009; Victora et al., 2016)

In a study published in *Archives of General Psychiatry* (Kramer et al., 2008), 17,046 infants enrolled in 1996 and 13,889 (82%) were followed up in 2005. In terms of outcomes, verbal IQ was 7.5 points higher with breastfeeding and full-scale IQ 5.9 points higher. On average, there was a higher total increase for boys of

8 points and 7 points for girls. Teacher academic ratings were also significantly better among the breastfed infants than the artificially-fed. These results were statistically cleansed to remove confounding factors, such as socioeconomic status.

What are Common MSK Problems of Newborns Struggling to Breastfeed?

Infants who fail to feed effectively may show:

» Torticollis/stiff neck/preferred head position

» TMJ dysfunction

» Difficulty latching due to muscular hypotonia or hypertonia

» Hypertonic gag reflex

» Tongue bundling

» Headache, sore neck, pain

A neonatal hospital unit in 1986 found that disturbed suck was related to intraventricular hemorrhage, length of labor, type of delivery, maternal anesthesia, low birthweight, low gestational age, barbiturates, and cocaine. Babies delivered by unplanned cesareans had a significant increase in total feeding time compared with babies delivered vaginally (Smith, 2007).

Babies from NICU environments may have had a negative experience with vfdoral stimuli—endotracheal, gavage tubes taped to face, multiple caregivers, etc. Tongue-tip elevation (tongue to hard palate that interferes with nipple insertion) is common in premature babies and babies with a low APGAR may demonstrate a poorer suck. Ways to feed these babies are found in the hospital setting. The babies who present to chiropractors are those who have left the hospital but still cannot sustain breastfeeding.

What Do Chiropractors Actually Do in this Population?

Chiropractors observe and check the following:

» Check rooting reflex.

» Check suck reflex. Place finger on baby's lower lip. If baby doesn't extend tongue to pick up finger, lay finger on anterior part of tongue. Check for strength of suck, number of beats of suck cycle, oral motor tone, endurance, coordination of Suck Swallow Respiration (SSR) rhythm.

» Check for tongue-tie.

» Check the palate, and the slope and shape of palate.

» Check for lateralization of the tongue.

» Check muscles used in suck.

» Check the use of the orbicularis oris.

» Check other structures involved in suck: TMJ, Hyoid, Infrahyoid muscles, Masseter, Pterygoid Temporalis, Frontal rooting reflex and gag reflex, Tongue tremors, tongue bundling, Buccal fat pads configuration with suck.

Linda Smith (2007) documented that the infants use 6 cranial nerves, 22 bones connecting at 34 sutures, and 60 voluntary and involuntary muscles in order to suck, swallow, and breathe.

Table 3: Cranial nerve review: Nerve, origin, action

Trigeminal(V)	Motor-Pons S-Trigeminal G.	Chewing Face Sensation
Facial (VII)	Motor-Pons S-Geniculate G.	Smile, Rooting, Taste Sensation
Glossopharyngeal (IX)	Motor-Medulla Sensory Ganglion	Taste, Gag Reflex, Swallowing
Vagus (X)	Same As IX	Taste, Speaking Cough
Hypoglossal (XII)	Nucleus-Medulla	Movements Of Tongue

What can go wrong?

» Mechanical forces on the cranium during birth can disrupt normal nerve function.

» Forceps over the parietal bone can cause bruising to cranial nerve V.

» Cranial Nerve VII is very superficial and can be easily compromised, affecting rooting, latching, and sucking responses.

Chiropractic Protocols for the Suboptimal-Feeding Infant

1. Symptoms

2. Signs

3. Safety

4. Subgrouping

5. Management

Symptoms of Suboptimal Feeding

Painful breastfeeding, misshapen nipples after feeding, damaged nipples (cracked, sores, bleeding), breast feels full after feed, mastitis, blocked ducts.

Noisy feeding (clicking), inefficient/slow feeding, constant feeding, chewing, and dribbling milk.

Signs of Suboptimal Feeding

Poor/slow growth (weight, length, head circumference), abnormal suck, high/anterior palate, restricted movement of tongue/jaw/palate/cervical spine, SCM tightness/hyper- or hypotonic muscles of mastication.

Safety Factors

Watch for the following:

> » Dehydration, poor weight gain, ANY weight loss, <6 wet diapers in 24 hours, sunken fontanelle, lethargy, etc.

» Failure to thrive: Insufficient growth (weight, then length, then head circumference), developmental delay

» Attachment to mother/parents : Difficulty with bonding

» Maternal depression, anxiety, and lowered quality of life: Feeding difficulties and postnatal depression are associated

» Subgrouping types of feeding dysfunction: These have been done in many ways. This is just a simple method that can help to categorize the problem, that, with treatment, should change over a short treatment period. We give ourselves a maximum of 10 days, as we cannot expect more from the family, and, if we have scoped the problem correctly, we should be able to treat and allow for healing within that timeframe.

Disorganized

Some degree of one or more of the following:

» Weak suck

» Inefficient/slow feeding at breast

» Postural preference affecting (but not preventing) feeding

» Discomfort for mother

~ Breastfeeding usually possible with resolution of MSK, and positioning and attachment support

Dysfunctional

Moderate degree of one or more of the following:

» Weak suck, may be dribbling

» Inefficient/slow feeding at the breast or bottle (limits breastfeeding)

» Postural preference limiting feeding

» Painful for mother

» Weight increasing but not optimally

~ May be unable to exclusively breastfeed unless the mother is very highly motivated and has time and resources to persist.

Disordered

Severe feeding difficulty that makes feeding a difficult time for baby or mother.

» Poor, ineffective suck that makes feeding from breast or bottle very difficult

» Unable to take a full feed from the breast

» Slow, dribbling feeding from a bottle

» Pain for mother prevents or cuts short breastfeeds

» Mastitis or blocked ducts at least once

» Significant nipple/areola damage

» No weight gain, or weight loss

» Unable to feed exclusively at the breast

» Struggles to feed from a bottle

Each of these three subgroups (disorganized, dysfunctional, disordered) may present with or without infant disinterest in feeding ("happy to starve"). Disinterest may complicate any of these three scenarios. It may coexist with any of these three groups or may be secondary to dysfunctional or disordered feeding, where the baby's internal cost/benefit analysis makes not feeding the better option (less exhausting). In a disordered-feeding baby, disinterest may create a serious situation. This can become the case where breastfeeding causes pain to the infant. A classic example of this is breastfeeding-induced headache.

A baby with a headache can be described as a baby who will show signs of hunger (but will seldom, if ever, cry for feeding), start to feed, then cry and pull back, then start the cycle again. They may also hold their head and show signs of discomfort (photo). Treat this by clearing any problems with the cervical spine (as there is a known mechanism) and through treating any pain-producing muscles of the scalp, such as temporalis and gala aponeurotica, as well as the cervical spine. This should take one treatment, two at most, and the problem should be solved.

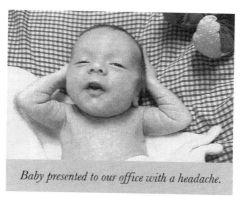

Baby presented to our office with a headache.

What is the Risk of Chiropractic Management of Feeding Disorders?

Chiropractic care has been repeatedly shown to have a good safety record in infant care (Todd, Carroll, Robinson, & Mitchell, 2016). There is, however, one very key sign that must be observed in any infant care, particularly in any baby with a feeding difficulty: dehydration. Extra attention is required to ensure that they are safe to receive treatment and do not require a different practitioner on that day. As infants are "small pitchers with large spouts" and are readily dehydrated, these cases require frequent monitoring for signs of dehydration. It is appropriate to discuss this with families, particularly in those infants who are disinterested in feeding or are in the more severe subgroups of dysfunctional or disordered feeding.

It is important to ask parents how many wet and dirty diapers they have each day. There must be more than six to feel assured that there is good input and thus, good output.

Growth should also be carefully monitored in any baby with a feeding difficulty. Newborns, after the normal loss of up to 10% of their weight, should start to gain about 1 oz (30 grams) per day. Weight, length, and head circumference are required to be measured and plotted on the infant's WHO growth chart. Slowing of weight gain, or any weight loss, is a high risk for dehydration. Slowing or halting of length and head circumference are signs of a severe or longer-standing feeding problem, or secondary underlying illness, including congenital anomalies. Head (brain) growth will be preserved ahead of all other measurements. Hence, problems in this area require particular attention. It may be a sign of malnutrition, or congenital condition, or other problems, including cranial synostosis. Every healthcare professional is responsible for updating an accurate growth chart and heeding the findings.

In any feeding problem, support and contextualized reassurance (where appropriate) should be provided for the parents. If there are MSK findings, this should be addressed rapidly while monitoring vital signs, including growth. If there is no improvement with MSK treatment, referral to appropriate breastfeeding support should be readily made. Concurrent care with International Board Certified Lactation Consultants should be standard.

For Disorganized-Feeding Problems

» Monitor weight, length, and head circumference.

» Monitor for dehydration and number of wet diapers.

» Provide support and contextualized reassurance to the mother or family.

» Address any MSK problems.

» If no improvement with MSK care, refer to breastfeeding support group or their midwife.

» Expect resolution or significant improvement with these measures.

For Dysfunctional-Feeding Problems

» Monitor weight, length, and head circumference.

» Monitor for dehydration (educate family to monitor).

» Provide support and contextualized reassurance to the mother or family.

» Suggest early involvement in breastfeeding support: Support groups, midwife, lactation consultant.

» Address any MSK problems.

» Assess or refer for assessment of tongue-tie (if painful feeding, noisy feeding, misshapen nipples after feeding).

» Consider the role of nipple shields, hand or pump expression, cup, or syringe, depending on the age of the infant and goals of the mother.

» The outcome often depends on how much the mother or family is able or willing to do.

~ Time and energy, expressing, cost of equipment, other children

For Disordered-Feeding Patterns

» Carefully and regularly monitor weight, length, and head circumference.

» Monitor for dehydration.

» Monitor mother and communicate with her (depression, anxiety, quality of life).

» Provide support and contextualized reassurance (if appropriate) to the mother or family. Refer mother for support, if required.

» Readily refer the infant or mother, if required.

» Suggest early involvement with breastfeeding support: Midwife or lactation consultant.

» Have a plan for supplementation (age dependent), and at what stage this would be implemented (preferably with lactation consultant input).

» Address any MSK problems.

» Assess, or refer for assessment of tongue-tie (if painful feeding, noisy feeding, misshapen nipples after feeding).

» Consider the role of nipple shields, hand or pump expression, cup, or syringe, depending on the age of the infant and goals of the mother.

» May be unable to feed exclusively at the breast. Support any breast milk transfer by age-appropriate means.

For Disinterested-Feeding Patterns

May coexist with any classification.

» May be primary (disinterest leading to difficulties).

» May be secondary (dysfunctional or disordered feeding creating a situation where feeding is too difficult for the infant to be worth trying).

» Will complicate any feeding picture.

» Warrants additional monitoring for growth, hydration, and development.

The balance between getting the baby sufficiently fed and dyad quality of life is difficult in these cases. Communication with the family, respecting the mother's opinion, and monitoring the clinical picture are key factors to balance. Refer to a pediatrician if lactation-consultant support has been unsuccessful. A board-certified lactation consultant should always be the first point of contact in these cases.

CHAPTER 9

Infant Postural Preferences and Musculoskeletal Dysfunctions

You won't find a chapter with this title in virtually any major pediatric textbook. This is interesting because musculoskeletal health and functional posture are important at any age. It is a key concept for chiropractors who are musculoskeletalists who deal with the problems in this system as their primary focus every day of their practicing life. Despite growing interest in the newborn spine and its possible damage during birth by manual therapists, obstetricians, pathologists, and neurologists (Ritzman, 2004), there is still very little research into the management of the problem when it develops.

Why Would Newborns Need a Musculoskeletal Assessment?

Musculoskeletal irritation and injury are common at all ages. Birth injury, unless major and life-threatening, is underrecognized and undertreated (Gottlieb, 1993). Birth, even under normal conditions, consists of significant traction and rotation of the baby's head, with sufficient force to cause clavicle fracture, and is known as "an unavoidable side effect of birth" in some vaginal births (Mavrogenis, Mitsiokapa, Kanellopoulos, Ruggeri, & Papageloupoulos, 2011). Birth injuries are more common when there are more birth interventions. Forceps deliveries are associated with skull fractures, cranial nerve palsies, brachial plexus injuries, facial nerve injuries, and torticollis (Ritzman, 2004).

Cephalohematomas and cranial fractures are associated with Ventouse (vacuum) delivery. Vacuum extraction has been shown to be a strong predictor of early cessation of breastfeeding due to injury (Hall, Chesters, & Robinson, 2002). It is increasingly common for births to be assisted with vacuum extraction equipment or surgery (Kozak & Weeks, 2002). In a study of 200 children presenting to a chiropractic clinic with pain and other physiologic disturbance, 95% demonstrated notable birth trauma (Edwards et al., 2010). In a much earlier and larger medical study (Frymann, 1966) of 1,250 newborns, 89% showed some mechanical strain or restriction.

Birth injuries are shown in box on page 87. Mild injuries are those that would likely only be detected by a musculoskeletal assessment. The list of moderate and severe injuries would likely be detected with the current early examination, which, in the UK, occurs within 72 hours of birth.

However, musculoskeletal injuries are not always detected. Joseph and Rosenfeld (1990) stated that the frequency of fractures diagnosed in the first assessment is significantly underestimated. One chiropractor in Norway (Monson, 2013) found 16 cases of undetected clavicle fractures from birth in a single practice. Forty-six rib fractures, occurring from, but undetected, at birth in 13 cases, have been reported in the literature (Van Rijn, Bilo, & Robben, 2009).

Another overlooked birth injury is torticollis. Torticollis is a wry neck resulting in the distorted position of the head due to an inability to utilize full cervical spine range of motion, almost always declared a birth injury at the neonatal stage (Cheng & Au, 1994). The incidence rate has been reported as being between 1.2% to 3.92% (Chen, Chang, Hsieh, Yen, & Chen, 2005; Cheng & Au, 1994). A more recent study found a much higher rate of 16% and suggested that this condition is frequently missed due to incomplete musculoskeletal examination (Stellwagon et al., 2008).

Other medical authors declare that missed diagnoses in infant pathology and neurology are high at 10% to 30% (Rossitch & Oakes, 1992; Towbin, 1964). Poor detection rates of early musculoskeletal injuries could be at least partly because medical clinicians may not feel comfortable with diagnosis and treatment of musculoskeletal injuries in childhood (Gill & Sharif, 2012; Jandial, Myers, & Wise, 2009). Perhaps that is part of the old story; if your only tool is a hammer, everything looks like a nail.

It seems logical that the general examination in hospitals is focused on the diagnosis of severe (life-threatening) types of trauma, and mild or moderate injuries may be overlooked. Birth is fundamentally a mechanical problem between the size of the head of the baby and the relative size of the pelvis of the mother. Birth was historically handled by the mother herself along with a "wise woman."

Around the end of the 17th century, there was a decline in women's knowledge (as a result of religious and church persecutions), followed by the birth (forgive the pun) of the male obstetrician. This brought about the invention of instruments of delivery, including the "iron hands of Palfijn" (1721), which was the first obstetrical forceps. A later version of forceps, developed by Christian Kielland (1871-1941), are still in use today. It has been shown in wide research that forceps delivery is a common etiology for birth injury.

High-risk births can, in a simplistic fashion, be categorized as:

1. arrested parturition (uncoordinated or weak labor caused by fear, pain, exhaustion, or induction),

2. extremely rapid delivery (due to immense power of contractions),

3. breech delivery (feet first) or,

4. delivery with a deflected head (spine to spine, with their head less able to bend during parturition).

These almost all require some medical assistance and sometimes multiple interventions. Interventions during birth that affect the cervical spine (that research has found is commonly involved) can be categorized as pressure from above, traction from below, and/or any rotary forces.

It is interesting to note that Leonardo da Vinci's accurate anatomical drawings of the gravid mother were all based on autopsies of mothers who died during childbirth, and all of the babies were in breech position. Now, breech position, particularly in the USA, is an indication for cesarean surgery.

Modern practices are better (probably) than ancient practices. Many people believe that birth is safe where modern obstetrical practices are used. Still, it is also important to note that, at the time of this writing, 18 August 2018, the USA has found its place as 46th in maternal mortality at, or around, the time of birth, meaning 45 countries are safer than the USA to give birth (*USA Today*, 2018).

Prevalence of neonatal birth injuries classified as mild, moderate, and severe.	
MILD	» Asymmetry of the head: 61% » Facial asymmetry: 42% » Torticollis: 16% » Asymmetry of the mandible: 13% » Nasal septum deviation: 0.93%
MODERATE	» Clavicle fracture: 0.4-10% » Facial nerve injury: 0.75% » Bruising and tearing of spinal nerve roots: 0.3% » Brachial Plexus: 0.11-0.26%
SEVERE	» Extra- and subdural hemorrhage into joint capsules, and torn ligaments and dura: 0.96% » Hemorrhages of vertebral arteries: 0.85%

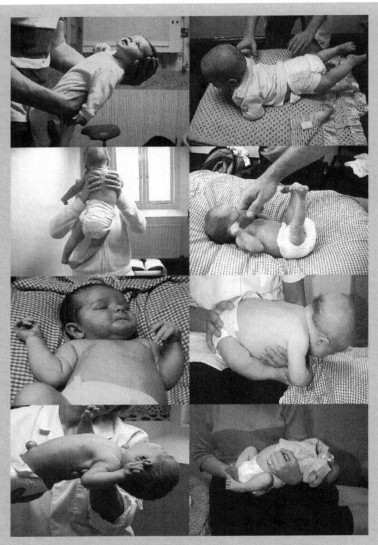

These pictures show typical cases of IISMO. The child often adopts an arched or other antalgic posture. Twisting of the upper body with respect to the pelvis can also be noted. In addition, the head may be rotated. Head rotation is often most noticeable when the child is placed in the supine position. Unilateral paraspinal muscle hypertonicity causes the baby to laterally flex the trunk to one side when lying down. Full flexion and lateral flexion are other choices to find comfort. (Reproduced from Open Access Journal of Clinical Chiropractic Pediatrics, *2005*). © *Joyce Miller, Photographer. All parents gave permission.*

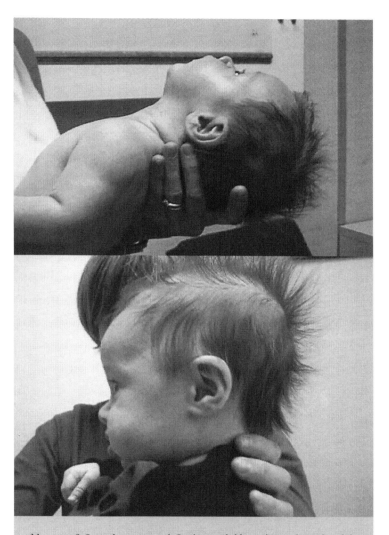

Neonate, 2.5 weeks, presented for inconsolable crying unless placed in extended position. The injury was to cervical and thoracic spine, due, most likely, to forceps delivery. The baby was treated and then able to attain an upright position with ease. The parents gave the novel explanation that because the baby extended his head back to look at the ceiling, that the baby "wanted to be an astronaut." This was a sweet interpretation of his musculoskeletal need to hold that position because it was his only position of comfort.

Who Presents to the Chiropractic Office?

Inconsolable, Irritable Infants

At increased risks of musculoskeletal injury, and thus, irritability, is the male child born to prima para mothers using assisted methods (Torvaldson et al., 2006). This is a very common patient whose parents present him to a chiropractor. The baby very often demonstrates a postural preference that has not always been previously recognized as characterized by discomfort.

A sample of those with strong postural preferences is shown in the photos below. These babies were presented as irritable infants. In our clinic, we have used the term Irritable Infant Syndrome of Musculoskeletal Origin to describe their strong preference for an antalgic posture to find their comfort level. Then, they cease crying. They cannot achieve normal posture.

Sleep Disorders

Another very common complaint in infants is sleep disturbances. The abnormal muscle tone seen in IISMO prevents the child from comfortably taking certain positions while in bed. Parents today are advised to have their babies sleep supine, but children with any hyperextended posture will not enjoy lying on their backs, as this forces the trunk into a neutral position, no doubt causing discomfort. As we have learned from parents who present their infants for care, their primary concern is the inability to sleep supine. This is appropriate because the Back-to-Sleep program has been developed to lower the risk for Sudden Infant Death Syndrome (SIDS) (AAP 1992; AAP, 2005). Of course, a risk of death outweighs a risk for discomfort. However, if the second causes the first, and there is a quick and safe therapy to alleviate the problem, this would be of interest to public health. Chiropractic care has been shown to allow babies who could not previously sleep supine in comfort to do so (Miller et al., 2018). This is a breakthrough in improving public health for the infant.

Public Health Supported by Chiropractors

Chiropractors should take a role in supporting the care of infants (as with all patients). There is an important role in not only helping neonate with problems with supine sleep but to alleviate breast-feeding problems (Miller et al., 2016), as well as crying problems, which is a leading cause of abuse in this age-group of children (Carbaugh, 2004). Solving these issues contributes to public health.

Postural Medicine

Although postural preferences in newborns have been the subject of study for some time (Casaer, 1979), whether these should be treated has been questioned (Rosenbaum, 2006). However, when left untreated, there is evidence (Binder, 1987; Boere-BooneKamp & van der Linden-Kuiper, 2001; Cioni, Ferrari, & Prechtl, 1989; Philiippi et al., 2006) of long-term persistence of postural asymmetries in up to 50% of cases. This is why researchers and clinicians highlighted the importance of therapeutic procedures, even in the early years of life. Postural fault concentrates stress locally, which sooner or later, may cause pain, discomfort, or further dysfunction.

Postural medicine studies the effects of position and gravity on the human body (Martin-Du Pau et al., 2004). For example, a patient with disc disease generally has more pain while seated. Sudden Infant Death Syndrome (SIDS) is more common in prone sleep (AAP, 1992). Gastroesophageal-reflux disease (GERD) may be alleviated by sitting upright.

Just as architects take into account the laws of gravity and weight distribution to increase resistance to stress and strains in a building under construction, the human body requires good alignment with a straight (uncurved) spine balanced over the lower limbs to distribute the weight evenly over discs, ligaments, and joints. Oddly, these principles are often overlooked in young infants, possibly because they do not stand upright.

Fortunately, chiropractors are not alone in recognizing the aberrant posture of the infant (see box below). These correlate with irritable-infant syndromes. It seems logical that very often, cases of musculoskeletal irritability have been linked to or even mistakenly identified as excessive crying of infancy or infant colic (Miller & Caprini Croci, 2005). Perhaps a better overarching categorization is that of Infant Pain Syndromes.

> *Types of postural preferences that are common co-occurrences of excessive crying or pain syndromes of infancy found in the literature.*
>
> » Molded-baby syndrome (Rosegger et al., 1992)
> » Seventh Syndrome (Mau, 1968)
> » Congenital-predilection syndrome (Pschyrembel, 1998)
> » Turned head adducted hip-truncal curvature (TAC) syndrome (Hamanishi & Tanaka, 1994)
> » Squint-baby syndromes (Fulford & Brown, 1976)
> » IISMO (Irritable Infant Syndrome of Musculoskeletal Origin) (Miller, 2005)
> » KISS (Kinematic Imbalance due to Suboccipital Strain) (Biedermann, 1995)
> » Torticollis (Chen et al., 2005; Cheng & Au, 1994; Stellwagon et al., 2008)
> » Facial asymmetry, strabismus, hip dysplasia, asymmetric foot position, head, or cranial asymmetries (Boere-Boonekamp, 2001)

Heiner Biederman coined the term KISS (for Kinematic Imbalance due to Suboccipal Strain) for infants who presented with a primary upper-cervical extension, and a second type that has a lateral component (Biedermann, 1992). Several clinicians have discovered the same syndrome and have coined different terms because it was not widely researched. In our clinic, we have termed it Irritable Infant Syndrome of Musculoskeletal Origin (IISMO), partly because it includes wider aspects of the MSK system in its etiology. Everyone who has discussed these postural aberrations has found that they are more common in infants with certain obstetrical procedures, such as prolonged labor or fetal malposition, which often require the use of forceps or suction extraction (Boere-Boonekamp, 2001). There is a similar association with positional head deformity (PHD), also called plagiocephaly. Until or unless the ICD-diagnostic coding system determines that one of these definitions can be termed a diagnosis, clinicians will make their own decisions on which term that they use in their practices. My PhD thesis, titled *Effects of Musculoskeletal Dysfunction in Excessive Crying Syndromes of Infancy*, discusses the importance of MSK assessment in the infant age group, and I am reconstituting part of it herein.

Newborns are fully capable of experiencing pain. It seems to be logical that the child assumes these postures, although appearing to be very uncomfortable, as an antalgic posture (or one maintained due to the pain of moving out of this posture). Sometimes these babies display what is called *Tactile Defensive* behavior, or not wanting to be touched, and this can be most noticeable in the areas or junctions that are at the root of the antalgic posturing. It is logical that this type of posturing can be more common in one or both twins, where there have been prenatal space issues. You can find the cause of these aberrant postures quite easily by taking a history of the pregnancy and birth. Take a good history and then go back and take an even more thorough history, so that you don't miss any details, and the mother understands that you wish to fully understand what she has gone through.

Infants Feel Pain

Infants feel pain and have the same pain-producing and detecting physiology as adults, with fewer of the modifying influences. Most researchers agree that pain in children has been too long ignored, partly because it is misunderstood. Published literature as late as 2006 (Buonocore & Bellieni, 2010) stated that infants do not feel pain. This has been debunked as yet another myth surrounding infant health. More current research into the epidemiology of children's pain (Johnston & von Baeyer, 2012) recognized that children have pain, a good deal is musculoskeletal in origin, that it causes a burden for both the child and family, that it often becomes persistent and chronic, and it is very difficult to measure across age groups and clinical conditions. Musculoskeletal pain is the most common reason for the referral of children to rheumatologists (McGhee, Burks, Sheckels, & Jarvis, 2002), and pain has usually become chronic by the time of referral. Clinicians often miss or minimize subtle neurophysiological dysfunctions (AAP, 2005).

Musculoskeletal Problems and Pain

Despite musculoskeletal disorders being the leading cause of pain and the second greatest cause of disability around the world today, according to the World Health Organization (WHO) (World Health Organization, 2012), the musculoskeletal health of infants has been inadequately studied. Musculoskeletal maladaptation in infants is defined as failure of the motor system to respond, or to respond aberrantly, to appropriate sensory stimuli, due to biomechanical fault (Ferreira & James, 1972; Prechtl et al., 1997; Reher et al., 2008).

Normal patterns are generated when the musculoskeletal system responds appropriately to the central nervous system that mediates sensorimotor integration of the environment and physiological demands. When the musculoskeletal system cannot respond to normal signals due to biomechanical compromise, then the infant's response to signals may be inappropriate, inefficient, ineffective, or aberrant. These responses become characterized as functional problems of infancy, and most commonly include excessive crying, inefficient sleep habits, and sometimes ineffective feeding (St. James-Roberts, 2008).

Parents usually seek help for these and other problems of infancy. In Europe, 52% of parents seek complementary and alternative medicine (CAM) for their children (Zuzak et al., 2013), and many more seek conventional medical help worldwide (Kemper, Vohra, & Walls, 2008). Mothers are the main decision-makers in healthcare and when taking a child to see a chiropractor (Carlton, Johnson, & Cunliffe, 2009). Mothers will seek care until they find an answer.

Little is known about the impact of musculoskeletal dysfunctions in infancy other than that they account for significant use of resources. While half the expenditure on adult healthcare can be attributed to musculoskeletal disorders (WHO, 2012), the cost in infancy is also high (Miller, 2013; Morris, St. James-Roberts, Sleep, & Gillham, 2001; McGhee et al., 2002).

Link of Infant Complaints to MSK Causes

The etiology of crying and sleeping problems of infancy is not known, not the least of which is because the infant is not in a position to say, for example, "it hurts here." It is reasonable and logical to link these problems to dysfunctional musculoskeletal habitus, by way of opportunities stemming from intrauterine constraint or a difficult birth, resulting in discomfort or pain (Biedermann, 1995; Papousek & von Hofacker, 1998). Although the child's expression is generally interpreted as excessive crying or infant colic, these problems have been termed medically unexplained symptoms (Bakal et al., 2009). But, they have both traditionally and more recently been characterized as pain syndromes of infancy (PSI) (Geertsma & Hyams, 1989; Gudmundsson, 2010; Romanello et al., 2013; Williams-Frey, 2011). Many authors call birth trauma routine and unavoidable but still suggest evaluation immediately after birth to detect problems early, which could serve to avoid long-term consequences, such as chronic pain syndromes (e.g., Stellwagen et al., 2008).

Most researchers agree that pain in children has been too long ignored, partly because it is misunderstood. More recent research into the epidemiology of children's pain (Johnston & von Baeyer, 2012) recognizes that children have pain, a good deal is musculoskeletal in origin, that it causes a burden for both the child and family, that it often becomes persistent and chronic, and it is very difficult to measure across age groups and clinical conditions. Musculoskeletal pain is the most common reason for the referral of children to rheumatologists (McGhee et al., 2002), and pain has usually become chronic by the time of referral. It's not reasonable to minimize babies' pain or say that they are "not in as much pain as they seem to be."

Some researchers have proposed that spinally mediated reflexes, caused by tactile stimulation causing pain sensations, are heightened in neonates due to lower thresholds (Fitzgerald & Beggs, 2001). However, the behavioral reaction to pain often used to evaluate the child's discomfort cannot be considered accurate, primarily because facial reactions develop slowly, advancing over time and age. Therefore, neonate and young infants may demonstrate a diminished physical reaction to pain, despite having an exaggerated physiological response (Fitzgerald & Beggs, 2001). This means that *babies feel more pain but express it less.*

Infant pain is a specialized topic, not only because infants are pre-verbal but also because of clinical difficulty in assessing and measuring pain, and acknowledging that infants can have pain without apparent or obvious injury (Finley et al., 2005), or the clinician's inability to do an assessment that is capable of finding the injury.

Even physiological measurements, such as heart, respiratory rates, and blood pressure, may not be useful in this age group, particularly in persistent pain or discomfort. Observation of infant behaviors of facial expression, cry, body movements, sleep patterns, and inconsolability have been found useful but may also be indicative of a stress response and not just pain. Understanding of infant pain is limited in part due to ethical issues that limit invasive investigations in children (Fitzgerald & Walker, 2009) and prohibit study.

The phenomenon of central sensitization, well-known in adults, has also been observed in infancy (Walker, Tochiki, & Fitzgerald, 2009). This was demonstrated in long-term changes in response to pain after a difficult Neonatal Intensive Care Unit (NICU) experience (Lidow, 2002). It is not a great leap to propose that neonates who are exposed to multiple stressors, including instrumental delivery and invasive procedures during the time that the architecture of pain sensitivity and processing are still "under construction," may develop pain behaviors that persist. This concept is supported by a study (Hermann, Hobmeister, Demirakca, Zohsel, & Flor, 2006) that illustrated an increased perceptual sensitization to pain 9 to 14 years after painful NICU experience in both pre- and full-term infants. In our own practice, we have found it necessary to find ways to desensitize toddlers to centrally sensitized pain syndromes.

What Are the Risks of Musculoskeletal Examination?

If early detection of birth injury is a benefit, what are the risks of early musculoskeletal assessment? The assessment is non-invasive, done only by hand, without instrumentation and performed completely within the family unit, displaying less force than a mother might employ with a pat on the back to aid digestion or burp the baby (Hawk et al., 2009). The early examination provides an opportunity for treatment before further dysfunction begins. There are no reports in the literature of any injury due to chiropractic examination of the infant or child (Humphreys, 2010).

The converse question also must be asked. What are the risks of not doing a musculoskeletal screen? Are there any short or long-term risks of unnoticed spinal or muscular distortion or fractures, for example, in the clavicles or ribs? Damage does not occur exclusively to physical tissues but also to neural programs that control movement patterns, protective postures, and general alignment. That is why early treatment is recommended: to work within the critical window before unused synapses are pruned to correct neural patterns. It can be said that the earlier that a basic skill is learned, the longer the consequences of its malformation. Any maladaptation can derail kinesiological development long-term or require much more extensive treatment later. This is why even minor signs of postural aberration should be treated (Miller & Clarens, 2000).

Asymmetry alone may not cause problems but may predispose the child to difficulty in adapting to normal physical movement, or to adopt movement errors. Functional problems of childhood will become hardwired in the nervous system if they are not ameliorated (Biedermann, 1995).

Further, there are known risks associated with the excessively crying infant, such as shaken baby syndrome (Carbaugh, 2004) and insecure infant attachment (Taylor, Atkins, Kumar, Adams, & Glover, 2005). In cases where excessive crying occurs due to occult birth injury, then those risks may be avoided through early detection and treatment. As a chiropractor may be able to detect and treat mechanical problems of the excessively crying infant (Miller et al., 2012), there may be potential for an assessment to take place soon after birth, before the excessive crying begins in earnest. It is documented (Gill & Sharif, 2012; Jandial et al., 2009) that pediatricians and other non-MSK specialists have a low estimation of their ability to manage musculoskeletal cases. The chiropractor's expertise is in the exact area where other clinicians have little, and it is reasonable to recommend musculoskeletal expertise for musculoskeletal maladies (Foster, Hartvigsen, & Croft, 2012; Murphy, Justice, Paskowski, Perle, & Schneider, 2011).

Age Discrimination

Saying that children do not have musculoskeletal dysfunctions could be viewed as age discrimination. Stating that children do not require care for their musculoskeletal disadvantages is to remain blind to the long-term consequences that musculoskeletal disability has on health. The benefits of early assessment require evidence. Therefore, cohort or other types of studies should be undertaken to investigate whether infants who have intervention sustain any lower risk for complaints of excessive crying or other maladies of infants or toddlers. One study (Miller & Phillips, 2009) suggests that there are long-term benefits for children with infant colic who are treated early.

Prevention is preferred to treatment. But when treatment is needed, manual therapy has shown promise of effectiveness for excessive crying (Hayden & Mullinger, 2006; Karpelowsky, 2004; Koonin, 2005; Miller et al., 2012; Wiberg et al., 1999). The question remains as to the plausible mechanism of such treatment techniques.

CHAPTER 10

Finding and Treating the MSK Problem in Infants: How Does It Work?

I f a musculoskeletal examination is in order, then musculoskeletal treatment may be appropriate. Even in adults, determining the exact source of pain can be difficult due to referred or mimicked pain (Murphy & Hurwitz, 2007). For example, it is wellknown that gallbladder pain refers to the shoulder. Through active and passive movement and orthopedic tests, it is usually possible for the clinician to determine whether the origin of the pain is local (in the shoulder and biomechanical) or distant (gallbladder and pathological) (Slaven & Mathers, 2010).

None of this precision is possible with the infant, who may not be able to recognize pain for what it is, nor can they point to it or undergo testing procedures to discriminate the cause of pain (as muscle tests require resistance, which the infant cannot comprehend or provide of their own volition). Consider that the child will usually cry with pain. In some cases, crying may make the pain worse. The child may discontinue crying, but show other types of pain behavior, such as antalgic posture. If caregivers are not particularly observant, they may miss the signs of discomfort.

Chiropractors seek to prevent disability by directing care toward good postural alignment, as well as treating mild joint dysfunction, which can lower the threshold to pain. The lowered threshold to pain is called sensitization. This means that the body is more sensitive to pain, not less. This has been shown (Hermann et al., 2006) to occur in newborns with difficult births and to be maintained in the system through to adolescence. Sensitized nociceptors can discharge spontaneously with any innocuous movement or even gentle touch (Seaman & Cleveland, 1999). It is logical to suppose that children become more comfortable when the cause of their skewed posture is found and treated through re-alignment of the joints. A more balanced posture is accompanied by a cessation in pain behaviors (antalgic posture and crying).

Chiropractic Techniques to Treat Infants: Do They Work?

Joint hypomobility (lack of useful motion) is seen in infancy and is a logical sequela to mild spinal trauma during birth or relative lack of mobility during the crowded last weeks of gestation. Chiropractic treatment (gapping of the joints) in this age group consists of positional therapeutics (such as stretching or decompression), or "press and hold," or "touch and hold" soft-tissue techniques, as there are no thrusts presented to the young spine, and most of the force is transmitted via soft tissues to the spine, not to the spine directly. Any association of treatment with a "cracking" sound (cavitation) is completely inappropriate for the infant patient. Nowhere is it clearer that infants are NOT small adults, and key aspects of care must be reconsidered for the infant patient (Hawk et al., 2009; Marchand, 2013). There should be no high force presented to the infant's spine.

It is plausible that soft tissue work involving light-to-moderate tactile pressure and muscular stroking techniques might decrease muscular spasms, improve circulation, reduce adhesions, re-align soft tissues, re-align joints, improve range of motion, increase relaxation, and thus, alleviate pain or discomfort (National Center for Complementary and Alternative Medicine, 2007).

Other research demonstrated that therapeutic massage disrupts the acute inflammatory process, reducing levels of serum creatine kinase, and decreasing muscle soreness after extensive eccentric usage of muscles (Smith et al., 1994). This type of muscular activity could occur during birth processes, causing injury and pain. Soft-tissue manual therapy has been shown to alter pain-producing acute inflammation and substance P levels in patients with known soft-tissue pain syndromes (Field, 2002; Smith et al., 1994).

Success in doing this has also been shown with specific joint compression and deep tactile distribution of touch-pressure (Farber, 1982). However, other questions arise as to what mechanism might reduce pain in the child when the mode of onset and the mechanical lesion is less clear. Are pain-expressive behaviors due to mechanical lesions when no other source (such as infection, causing systemic markers) can be discerned? Could anything other than restored biomechanical comfort to the infant account for the change in behavioral patterns? Is mechanical force simply one potential key to unlock a complex physiological response that results in significant or profound pain modulation through the central nervous system (CNS)? Is pain connected to an emotional reaction? Virtually all adults have experienced aches and pains that can incite lowered patience and "shorten a fuse." In other words, physical pain may lead to irritability, or upset of the nervous system and the emotions.

One of the hallmarks of the inconsolable baby is a hyperactive autonomic nervous system (ANS) (LaGasse, Neal, & Lester, 2008) that has two components: the sympathetic and parasympathetic nervous systems (SNS and PNS, respectively). It is reasonable that inconsolable crying is related to a hyperactive sympathetic nervous system (SNS), and this has been described in both baby and caregiver (LaGasse et al., 2008). The cry is like a siren to the parent, an aversive stimulus, which must be turned off. When the cause cannot be found (and thus, relieved), the parent becomes as tense as the child. Several studies (Miller & Newell, 2012; Murray, 1979; St. James-Roberts, 1999) have shown correlations between the baby's inconsolability and the mother's report of stress. It is likely that these tensions then reinforce each other, creating an increasing imbalance in the autonomic nervous system. Treatment may be required to rebalance the system.

Manual Treatment to Reduce Pain

Studies in animals and adults have described a mechanism of chiropractic manual treatment as related to the gapping of zygapophysial joints, thus breaking adhesions that develop with hypomobility and stiffness of joints (Colloca, Keller, & Gunzburg, 2004). Pandiculation is a rigidness from hypomobility, a tendency of early stage stiffness documented in infancy (Philippi et al., 2006). This further suggests that musculoskeletal disorders that plague adults start early, as the presence of musculoskeletal imbalance at birth has been documented (Stellwagon et al., 2008; Wall & Glass, 2006).

How Does Manual Treatment Work?

How does it happen that a baby with inconsolable crying, who is treated by a chiropractor with manual therapy immediately, stops crying and becomes, in the words of the parent, a "completely changed" and placid baby?

Is this a biomechanical, physiological, structural change response that is too minor to be perceived by the parent or is it a powerful hyperalgesic dampening effect induced by the manipulation? Something in the baby's world has shifted. Is this a resetting of the autonomic nervous system? Hipperson (2004) proposed this theory and likened it to restarting a computer to put its actions back into balance, improving equipoise between inhibition and excitation.

Or, does a mechanical force to the painful tissue expedite a reduction in pain mediated by and resulting in a calmed ANS? Most of the medicine consists of chemical treatment. Chiropractic manual therapy is mechanical treatment but may involve a release of pain-busting chemicals with joint motion (Bialosky et al., 2009). Target tissues of manual therapy are a skeletal system, nervous system, and soft tissues. A mechanical force initiates a chain of neurophysiological responses that produce the outcomes. Mechanism of action is mediated by the dorsal horn of the spinal cord and periaqueductal gray zone.

Spinal cord responses following manual therapy provide a barrage of input to the CNS (acting as a counterirritant), documented with fMRI, resulting in a decreased activation of the dorsal horn (and accounting for analgesic effects of manipulation).

A supraspinal response, associated with ANS responses, results in descending inhibition of pain due to associated changes in the opioid system. Significant declines in serum levels of cytokines have been observed after manual therapy (Bialosky et al., 2009).

The same general effect is seen with another effective therapy for infant crying. Dicyclomine is a drug that decreases crying in colicky infants but has been removed from the market because of dangerous side effects of central nervous suppression and death (Garrison & Christakis, 2000). Its ability to resolve crying indicates nothing about the cause of the condition, as it is a central nerve depressant with side effects of coma and death. Thus, its effects are general, not specific to the cause of colic. It appears that changes to the entire system are mediated by the central nervous system, whether these changes are instituted chemically or mechanically.

Fortunately, when CNS changes are incited through mechanical stimulation, adverse effects are extremely unlikely. The mechanism of therapy may depend on whether it is a "hardware" or "software" type of problem. Therefore, two mechanisms are proposed.

Proposed Mechanisms of Manual Therapy In Infants

Two parallel mechanisms of healing in children with manual therapy are proposed herein. The first is simple biomechanical realignment, by skilled hands, of joints misaligned by intrauterine constraint or difficult birth. The second is due to nervous system changes through biomechanical reconfiguration, allowing relief of an anatomical irritation; this may be coupled with CNS chemical and neurological pain desensitization. These mechanisms could work separately or in tandem.

First, in some patients, there are biomechanical faults: a shortened muscle through fibrosis; a damaged ligament, such as the anterior talofibular ligament in a sprained ankle; or a loosened (or frozen) spinal joint caused by a difficult birth process. When these are corrected, it is like screwing the lid onto a jar. When it is aligned correctly, the system works well but when it is misaligned, the cover cannot be replaced tightly, and the system never works flawlessly until corrected. Sometimes, mechanical fault is simply a matter of re-alignment, and this can be treated by skilled therapy with almost instant relief for the patient (with some time for healing to take place, depending on the time frame and degree of the injury). With good alignment comes improved comfort. This is primarily a local phenomenon. Treatment works immediately and effectively. This is when the parents say, "he is like a completely different baby," and they cannot stop singing your praises after just one treatment, when the therapy was, in fact, a straightforward biomechanical correction for an experienced chiropractor.

Second, the human body also works as a complex unit. There are central (brain) mechanisms that assist in pain reduction, such as descending inhibitory impulses. This is thought to be inhibited in infants, relative to adults. However, without joint re-alignment, the pain reduction may be only temporary, and it may have to be instituted repeatedly until the body adopts a new pain-free or irritant-free status quo. The system resets. This can occur instantaneously, or it can take time, over a few sessions, for the system to adapt to the change. Frequent treatment "reminds" the body to maintain appropriate alignment until full recovery or normal elasticity of the tissues ensue. The CNS "resets" through a series of neurological and chemical cascades (Bialosky, Bishop, Price, Robinson, & George, 2009). Our research has shown that the average number of treatments required is four, with the most common number being three. Certainly, there are many cases where the change came after the first treatment. However, parents return because they cannot believe that the change could have occurred so quickly, and also, feared recurrence if they do not seek more care. This is parent-driven care instead of clinician-driven care.

The question remains as to why children recover more quickly than adults. Of course, young tissue heals faster. Newborn babies have stem cells that can regenerate into any other kind of cell. Also, there is less (if any) psychological overlay in the child, and there is no reason for the child to have sickness behavior or an aversion to wellness. There is no reinforcement for staying ill for an infant, as there may be with a teen or adult. It is unlikely that there is any attention to positive reinforcement of illness behavior during infancy. It is more likely that the time it takes to reset the system is not accounted for by hesitance in the psychology of the child but rather, time for the system to rebalance or heal after some time out of equilibrium. The earlier effective treatment occurs, the less likely the organism is to become sensitized. The earlier it happens, the less time it takes for realignment and the ability to sustain appropriate posture to manifest. The key is to return the child to pain-free full function. The child may then feel better, feed better, sleep better, and cry less. When functions improve, their behaviors tend to improve. It stands to reason that removing the irritant could have long-term, as well as short-term, benefits.

These two mechanisms may help explain why some babies improve instantaneously with one manipulation, while others require a series of treatments (most commonly three, but on average, four) recovering more slowly, but still over a shorter period than the known natural history of the disorder (Miller et al., 2012; Wolke et al., 2002).

How Does this Reflect Modern Chiropractic Care?

The chiropractic profession has embraced the evidence-based model. Long gone are the days when the fundamentalist chiropractic profession believed in manipulation as a panacea for all of humanity's ills, reliant upon Palmer's (1910) ideas that blockage (subluxation) of a certain lifeforce was a primary cause of illness. The chiropractic profession subscribes to Engel's proposed (1977) biopsychosocial model (Fava & Sonino, 2008) of health and disease that embraces a multifactorial cause of disease or disorders (biological, psychological, social). For infants, another model may be more appropriate for musculoskeletal disorders and pain comprising components of mechanical, chemical, and central sensitivity (Breen, 2013) and a lesser emphasis on the psychological and social domains.

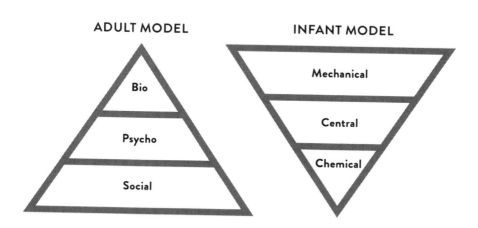

These figures show comparisons of models of illness in adults versus infants.

The chiropractic profession also supports public health measures, particularly those that relate to spinal health. Chiropractors see their role as caring for and preventing musculoskeletal problems as parallel to that of podiatrists taking care of foot problems, or dentists caring for teeth. They apply these principles to all age groups. Although there is plenty of empirical evidence that it works for their patients, there is still a need for higher levels of evidence. There is, however, evidence that treatment is safe.

CHAPTER 11

Safety of Chiropractic Care for Infants

A colleague from the local hospital told me why she referred dozens, if not hundreds, of babies to our clinic; "you may not help every baby, but you will not hurt any baby." She pointed out that treatment is mild low-force touch to a restricted barrier, which did not provide significant enough force to cause injury. But does research show that chiropractic care is safe for infants?

When a child is presented for healthcare, parents, the family, healthcare providers, and society presume it is safe. Safety is the bedrock upon which all healthcare is based. After all, the first rule is, "Do no harm." Safety for all patients is under scrutiny, and the pediatric population is particularly vulnerable because they cannot speak for themselves. Further, parents are equally vulnerable, as they are emotionally involved and may not be able to regulate their stress, let alone that of their child. Parents may have difficulty making decisions for their child and will hand treatment decisions over to the clinician. The clinician must take responsibility for the safety of the child under treatment.

Safety is a chief concern in all of pediatric healthcare. For example, the safety of medications given to children is increasingly considered an important public health issue (Vernacchio, Kelly, Kaufman, & Mitchell, 2009). Common remedies, such as cough and cold medications for children, are no longer routinely recommended because of negative side effects (Sharfstein, North, & Serwint, 2007). The National Patient Safety Agency in the UK has tracked safety incidents in pediatric patients and reported many concerns (Stephenson, 2007). Reviewing 33,446 reports on pediatric care in 2006, they found that 19% of children in care experienced medication problems. Other breaches of safety include 14% procedure problems, 9% errors in documentation, and 7% errors in clinical assessment, among other incidents. Of particular concern was the rate of medication error in children (19%) versus that in adults (9%) (Stephenson, 2007). The use of medication in children is common. A 2009 report found that the majority of U.S. children less than 12 years of age use one or more medications weekly (Vernacchio et al., 2009). Half of the infants in our study were, or had been on medications when they presented to our clinic.

There is a trend showing that parents often seek complementary and alternative medicine (CAM) for their children (Black et al., 2015; Kemper, Vohra, & Walls, 2008). Chiropractic (and manual therapy, in general) is the most common alternative care sought by parents for their child (Black et al., 2015). Choosing a drug-free profession may reinforce the conjecture that parental choice of alternative care for their child may be partly due to "fear of pharma," or phobia related to the use of pharmacology, particularly glucocorticoids (Hon et al., 2006).

Safety could be the main reason that parents turn to complementary and alternative medicine (CAM) therapies (Hon et al.,

2006). However, parents may seek a wide variety of practitioners and chiropractors may be just one of several clinicians treating a child. Data collection of 2,033 pediatric cases that presented to the AECC teaching clinic between 2000 and 2006 showed that over 90% had seen other clinicians and most had seen multiple types of practitioners for the same condition (Miller, 2009). It is unlikely that chiropractic would be the first choice of clinician, and traditionally, it was most likely far down the line. However, having worked in a busy chiropractic pediatric practice in 2018, I can say that more and more parents are thinking of chiropractors early rather than later for children, as there is an understanding that when the problems are pain, discomfort, or movement disorders, manual therapy may be the first choice.

Among manual therapists, chiropractors are registered, recognized, and one of the top three healthcare clinicians. This may be because chiropractors are the first choice for parents who utilize manual therapy for their infant. However, that is purely an observation of mine, and further research is required to find the actual motivation for parents to take their child to chiropractors. The fact is that they do, and they do it in large numbers, often having been referred by other healthcare practitioners, in our clinic at least 60% to 80% of the time, depending on the condition (Miller et al., 2009; Miller et al., 2018).

The medical profession has long been aware that parents seek multiple types of healthcare for their children. McCann and Newell (2006) registered concern that children treated by herbs and other ingested remedies could have a reaction because of the (unknown) combination with pharmaceuticals medically prescribed. They further suggested that the complementary therapies (particularly physical therapies, such as massage and chiropractic) were less likely to interfere with biomedical treatment than complementary medicines that were ingested. Likewise, chiropractors must be aware of pharmaceuticals or other treatments undertaken by our patients, which might cause side effects or otherwise complicate our therapy.

In our clinic, we wrote a case report showing medication side effects that were the main affliction of a baby presented for our care (Holmes & Miller, 2014). This stresses the importance of a good history and knowing what medications the baby is already taking. Use of medication was found to be common in babies who presented for care in our pediatric practice. About half of the infants who presented were on medications, and often more than one and up to seven (Miller et al., 2016).

The purpose herein was to put together the research on the safety record of chiropractic care for children. Most safety research has been done on manual therapy done by multiple types of practitioners, not necessarily specialists, like chiropractors. It has been shown that manual therapy for children done by a chiropractor is 20 times less likely to result in an injury than that provided by a medical practitioner (Koch et al., 2002; Miller 2009). The type of care most commonly provided by chiropractors is spinal manipulative therapy (SMT). In our practice, we call this Pediatric Manual Therapy (PMT) to reflect the fact that the treatment has been greatly modified to respect the age, size, and development of the youngest patients.

The procedures that are modified in terms of amplitude, force, speed, and depth to the age-specific anatomy of the child, and delivered by chiropractors was the focus of the most recent prospective study of safety in chiropractic care for children. This study was carried out in the UK and studied the patients in 16 clinics that provided exclusive chiropractic care for infants. The mothers determined whether there were any adverse events or side effects that were caused by the chiropractor in the care of their infant. This is the best type of research to do, prospective, meaning while the care is being provided. It then is independent of the mother's memory, as she can declare right away if there were any problems with the care.

Further, the data were collected completely anonymously, so the mother could reveal exactly what she wanted to say, without concern for the perception of the doctor or anyone that she may strive to please. This precaution was taken because there is something called the "Halo effect." This implies that a patient or parent may wish to please the doctor or caregiver, and exaggerate the quality of the care when the doctor can overhear or see their opinions.

In 2,001 cases, no adverse event was reported. In total, 5.8% of the mothers reported a side effect, which were listed as mild and short in duration (less than 24 hours), and that required no additional care. These were described as irritability or increased tiredness after treatment and improved sleep. These were followed by being much better the next day. This is the best study so far because it was done prospectively with a large infant-patient base (Miller et al., 2018). In this large prospective study, chiropractic care was safe for infants. Other studies have been previously done. All show that the care is safe, with severe side effects rarely observed.

Side effects can be divided into three categories: mild (transient and requiring no healthcare), moderate (requiring additional healthcare), or severe (requiring hospital care). All three types of side effects were reported in the literature. Mild side effects were the most common.

Mild side effects secondary to chiropractic manipulation were found in two reports. One was a survey of parental report and one a retrospective record review, of a total of 1,076 pediatric patients having 8,290 treatments resulted in less than 1% experiencing irritability, soreness, or stiffness, all transient and requiring no additional care (Miller & Benfield, 2008).

Mild side effects secondary to manipulation delivered by medical doctors have also been reported. The rate of side effects was higher when manipulation was given by non-chiropractors. Two citations reported side effects from 600 children and 695 children, respectively, who were treated with "chiropractic therapy," but manipulation was performed by medical doctors (Biederman, 1992; Koch et al., 2002). These are included because they specifically describe the treatment as chiropractic therapy, although it was not delivered by chiropractors. In the first instance, there were no negative side effects, and in the second, there were effects of bradycardia, flush, and apnea, all of which subsided in 6 to 13 seconds.

Two points need to be made about the Koch (2002) research: 1) the "chiropractic" adjustments given to these infants were described as ranging between 30 and 70 Newtons (N) with an average of 50 N. 2) These side effects occurred preferentially ($p=0.0017$) in the youngest age group (<3 months). These side effects were considered as mild (transient) and occurred at a rate of 6% (84 out of 1,295 children) when combining both reports. It should be noted that this report regarded these as routine byproducts of treatment rather than negative side effects. That said, if in our chiropractic practice, there were a side effect of apnea in a child without this condition, this would be considered a negative side effect.

There is likely a difference in the severity of side effects that can be tolerated by medical providers than chiropractors, who operate much more conservative practices. Further, and the most important point here, is that treatments given by chiropractors to this age group (less than 3 months of age) use 15 to 35 times

LESS FORCE than the treatments Koch described. The high forces used by the medical clinicians are not required and are not indicated for this age group (Hawk, Schneider, Vallone, & Hewitt, 2016; Marchand, 2013).

The literature also reported moderate side effects secondary to chiropractic manipulation. Two moderate cases were reported that involved severe headache, stiff neck, and acute lumbar pain. These were treatments given by chiropractic students as part of a clinical trial (Vohra, Johnston, Cramer, & Humphreys, 2007).

Severe side effects secondary to chiropractic manipulation were extremely rare (4 in 41 years), and all occurred more than a quarter century ago. There were four citations in the systematic review, which resulted in severe side effects from chiropractic care of pediatric patients (Vohra et al., 2007).

In a 1978 case, a 7-year-old child had repeated trauma from midair somersaults landing on his cervical spine and occiput. The "chiropractor diagnosed cervical misalignment and initiated a course of rapid manual rotations of the head from side to side with flexion and hyper-extension" (Zimmerman, Kumar, Gadoth, & Hodges, 1978). The child became ill with vomiting, severe headache, and facial weakness. After two weeks, the child was released from the hospital and experienced persistent right-sided dysmetria with reduced quadrantanopia (blindness in the visual field) as long-term effects. As tragic as this case is (and it most certainly is), the child was also seen by a neurologist who did not suggest stopping either the gymnastics nor the manual therapy. Also, no known chiropractic treatment can be described as a rapid manual rotations side to side with flexion and extension. In short, this case is an aberration in routine presentations and therapies, and can be appropriately put to bed as a very unfortunate circumstance that has not been fully explained, other than by a pre-existing condition that was missed by all of the healthcare professionals, including the GP, neurologist, and chiropractor.

In 1992, a report of a chiropractic manipulation of a month-baby with torticollis had a serious long-term effect, resulting in quadriplegia regressing to paraplegia 18 months after treatment (Shafir & Kaufman, 1992). This occurred because infiltration of astrocytoma was unknown at the time of initial treatment. This was a case of a missed diagnosis by all of the healthcare providers who had seen the child. Another severe event occurred in 1983, with manipulation of a 12-year-old with osteogenesis imperfecta (a condition in which manipulation is contraindicated), resulting in paraplegia (Vohra et al., 2007).

In another event, chiropractic treatment in 1959 of a 12-year-old girl for neck pain persisting from congenital torticollis resulted in unsteady gait, decreased coordination, drowsiness, and neck pain, and hospitalization followed treatment (Vohra et al., 2007). Congenital occipitalization was diagnosed in the hospital. The correct diagnosis was missed by all of the clinicians who saw the child, an unfortunate circumstance.

Indirect adverse effects of treatment, including delayed medical treatments were also reported in the Vohra review. Nineteen cases were reported over 57 years (1940 to 1997). Sixteen cases involved delayed treatment and no serious adverse results occurred. These 16 cases were reported between 1992 and 1997. Three cases that developed serious adverse events occurred between 1940 and 1969. It seems that some learning has taken place in that there have been no severe adverse events in the chiropractic practice of children for many, many years. Any adverse event, however, is very unfortunate and must be learned from so that they can be prevented in the future.

Overall, the published evidence suggests that chiropractic care for the pediatric patient is low risk. The most thorough systematic review (Vohra et al., 2007) uncovered only eight incidents of hurt or harm to children due to chiropractic manipulation in 59 years (1940 to 1999), when billions of such treatments were given. The number needed to harm (**NNH**) has been calculated at one major neurovascular harm for every 250 million treatments. There are virtually no lawsuits or judgments of harm for children against chiropractors.

A more recent systematic review of adverse events after manual therapy found 31 reported cases of injuries from various healthcare providers (7 chiropractors, 1 medical practitioner, 1 osteopath, 2 physical therapists, and 1 unknown practitioner), 12 presented with serious injuries, where an underlying pre-existing pathology was identified (Todd, 2014). Three deaths were reported from a physical therapist, a craniosacral therapist, and an unknown practitioner. The current literature outlined no deaths associated with chiropractic care following manual therapy. This review stresses the importance of thorough history, examination, and imaging, if necessary, to rule out any potential pathology and congenital anomaly before applying manual therapy. They concluded that spinal manipulation remains a non-invasive, low-risk, therapeutic approach with minimal side effects.

Any adverse event is regrettable and provides lessons to be learned. There appears to be a pattern wherein early cases (as long as 70 years ago) had worse outcomes than more recent cases. This may indicate that some enlightenment has occurred in our profession over the years. Patients are no longer treated in a vacuum but are referred when it is clear that our care is not efficacious. Chiropractors are conscious that therapy must be effective before the natural decline of the disorder. Children usually respond quickly and generally do not require a course of treatment to extend beyond 2 to 3 weeks, unless complicating factors are present. It is important that the treatment shows evidence of improved outcomes in that timespan. If progress is not seen after two or three weeks of care, the clinician must reflect on the clinical usefulness of the approach and refer the patient for consultation with an appropriate specialist. The modern chiropractor is trained to recognize red flags and differential diagnoses, and this is reflected in the fact that no adverse events have been reported since 1992.

There are clear gaps in the dataset, with few studies of patient safety or adverse effects of chiropractic care. This may be a result of underreporting. Adverse effects should be reported as a part of normal routine practice. That is why prospective studies, undertaken in routine practice, are beneficial. Treatment is appropriate when using the safety/effectiveness matrix.

In the safety/effectiveness ratio, a therapy is appropriate if it has been shown to be both safe and effective. This is the case for chiropractic treatment in infant colic or excessive crying of infancy. In cases where there is insufficient evidence of effectiveness, but the therapy is safe, then a trial of treatment is appropriate. This is relevant to cases of poor infant breastfeeding, poor sleep, or other common complaints of infants. Parents should try all safe options to help their infant, and alleviate their own suffering, as these conditions are very hard on parents, as well as the baby.

Therefore, in cases where care has not yet been shown to have a positive effect, but the treatment has a good safety record, it is appropriate to undergo what is called a therapeutic trial. This is most appropriate in clinical situations where there are no known effective treatments with good safety records. For example, in dysfunctional breastfeeding, there is no proven treatment. However, chiropractic has been shown to be safe, with some evidence (though inconclusive) of good effect, so treatment is appropriate. A therapeutic trial should be undertaken for babies in pain, where other healthcare has not been helpful. A baby's pain must be respected and appropriately managed for relief. Safe management is a hallmark of low-impact, conservative, chiropractic care.

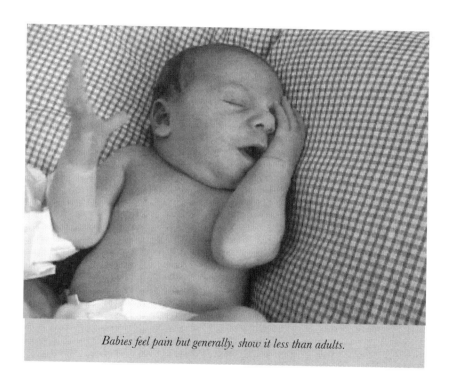

Babies feel pain but generally, show it less than adults.

Ways to Stay Safe

What is implicit in safe practice is the ability to identify risk and to modify treatment, taking that risk into account. There are too few incidents reported to ascertain where safety incidents cluster. That said, virtually all of the severe sequelae from misdiagnosis or treatment stemmed from the lack of recognition of occult pathology.

Non-recognition of pathology in a child increases the risk of a breach in safety under our care, as the child will be less resilient, as well as the fact that our care is inappropriate. Vigilance is required to detect occult pathology in every patient, although red flags may be more easily detected in adults who can speak for themselves and describe symptoms better than in children. Even if the infant has been seen by another health professional, a full assessment for pathology is still in order, prior to treatment.

The busy chiropractor may have questions; how should I interpret this evidence for my practice? Should I be concerned about the few incidents that have occurred? How can I lower the risk of adverse events in this patient group in my practice?

Chiropractors can look at practice through risk-reducing lenses and keep in mind some key points.

> » Know your limits. This is one of the keys of the Hippocratic Oath. Do not practice beyond your capabilities.

> » Continue to update skills in examination, treatment, notetaking, communication, equipment, resuscitation, and pediatric life support.

> » Do a thorough history and examination. Collect sufficient data to enable you to make a cogent decision on risk reduction.

> » Identify red flags and refer whenever indicated. Monitor every newborn for dehydration.

> » Always take vital signs before any treatment commences, and again at the end of treatment so that you know that the infant is healthy when leaving the premises.

» Always use the risk/benefit and risk/effectiveness ratios to determine the appropriateness of care. If the condition being treated does not have a clear efficacious therapy, do a therapeutic trial with a short course of treatment to determine whether benefits accrue more quickly than the natural history of the disorder. Always refer if good outcomes do not occur quickly.

» Use the correct technique for the age and condition of the patient, as outlined in best practice recommendations.

» Patients with comorbidities or medical needs should be co-managed with the appropriate health professional.

» Promote and support research.

» Keep thorough medical records.

» Report side effects and safety incidents so that data can be collected prospectively. Prospective reporting of all patient safety incidents is recommended and available. In the UK, the Chiropractic Reporting and Learning Systems (CRLS) is an online, anonymous system that accepts all types of patient safety events, including errors, accidents, mishaps, near-misses, or any deviation from the norm (Thiel & Bolton, 2006). The anonymity and security of the system encourage reporting from all chiropractors. This will result in accurate reporting of incidents for patients, as well as learning and feedback for the profession.

Conclusions based on the published literature demonstrate that manipulation, when given by a skilled chiropractor with years of training, carried out with low forces recommended for pediatric care, has few side effects in the healthy infant and child, and their recorded incidence is exceedingly low. Prospective evidence reported by mothers of infants undergoing care reported no adverse events and fewer than 5% reported side effects of short duration (less than 24 hours), consisting of irritability or restlessness. Positive side effects mothers reported included improved sleep.

Nothing is of greater importance in pediatric practice than taking a proactive stance to incorporate safe practice strategies into daily practice, and to report any incidents with the goal of safety and protection for all patients.

References

Alcantara, J., Ohm, J., & Kunz, D. (2009). The safety and effectiveness of pediatric chiropractic: A survey of chiropractors and parents in a practice-based research network. *Explore, 5*(5), 290-295.

American Academy of Pediatrics Task Force on Infant Sleep Position and Sudden Infant Death Syndrome. (1992). Positioning and SIDS. *Pediatrics, 89*(6), 1120-1126.

American Academy of Pediatrics Task Force on Sudden Infant Death Syndrome. (2005). The changing concepts of sudden infant death syndrome: Diagnostic coding shifts, controversies regarding the sleeping environment, and new variable to consider in reducing risk. *Pediatrics,* 116(5) 1245-1255; DOI: 10.1542/peds.2005-1499

American Academy of Pediatrics Subcommittee on Chronic Abdominal Pain. (2005). *Pediatrics, 115*(3), 812-815.

Bakal, D., Steiert, M., Coll, P., Schaefer, J., Kreitzer, J., & Sierpina, V. (2009). Teaching physicians, nurses and mental health professionals about medically unexplained symptoms. *Explore, 5*(2),121-124.

Barr R. G., Kramer M. S., Boisjoly C., McVey-White L., & Pless IB.(1998). Parental diary of infant cry and fuss behaviour. *Archives of Diseases of Childhood, 63,* 380-387.

Becker, K., Holtmann, M., Laucht, M., & Schmidt, M.H. (2004). Are regulatory problems in infancy precursors of later hyperkinetic symptoms? *Acta Paediatrica, 93,* 1463-1469.

Bialosky, J.E., Bishop, M.D., Price, D.D., Robinson, M.E., & George, S.Z. (2009). The mechanism of manual therapy in the treatment of musculoskeletal pain: A comprehensive model. *Manual Therapy, 14,* 531-538.

Biedermann, H. (1992). Kinnematic imbalance due to suboccipital strain in newborns. *Journal of Manual Medicine, 6,* 151-156.

Biedermann, H. (1995). Manual therapy in newborn and infants. *Journal Orthopedic Medicine, 12*(17), 2-9.

Biedermann, H. (2006). Manual medicine of functional disorders in children. *Medical Veritas, 3,* 803-814.

Binder, H., Eng, G.D., Gaiser, J.F., & Koch, B. (1987). Congenital muscular torticollis: Results of conservative management with long-term follow-up in 85 cases. *Archives Physical Medicine and Rehabilitation, 68*, 222-225.

Black, L.I., Clarke, T., Barnes, P.M., Stussman, B.J., & Nahin, R.L. (2015). Use of complementary health approaches among children in the United States: National Health Interview Survey 2007-2012. *National Health Status Report, 78*, 1-19.

Bodger, K., Ormerod, C., Shackcloth, D., & Harrison M., (2014). Development and validation of a rapid generic measure of disease control from the patient's perspective: The IBD-Control questionnaire. *Gut, 63*(7), 1092-1102.

Boere-Boonekamp, M.M., & van der Linden-Kuiper, L.T. (2001). Positional preference: Prevalence in infants and follow-up after two years. *Pediatrics, 107*, 339–343.

Bredart, A., Marrel, A., & Abetz-Webb, L. (2014). Interviewing to develop Patient-Reported Outcome (PRO) measures for clinical research: Eliciting patient's experience. *Health Quality of Life Outcomes, 12*, 12-15.

Breen, A.C. (2013). Low back pain: Identifying sub-groups. Clinical prediction rules and measuring results. *Proceedings of the World Federation of Chiropractic's 12th Biennial Congress*, Durban, South Africa.

Brod, M., Tesler, L.E., & Christensen, T.L. (2009). Qualitative research and content validity developing best practice based on science and experience. *Quality of Life Research, 18*(9), 1263-1278.

Bromfield, L., & Holzer, P. (2008). A national approach for child protection – Project Report Commissioned by the Community and Disability Services Ministers' Advisory Council. In National Child Protection Clearinghouse (Ed.) Australian Government Department of Families CSaiA, editor. Canberra, Australia Institute of Family Studies.

Browning, M., & Miller, J. (2008). Comparison of the short-term effects of chiropractic spinal manipulation and occipito-sacral decompression in the treatment of infant colic: A single-blinded, randomized, comparison trial. *Clinical Chiropractic, 11*(3), 122-129.

Buonocore, G., Bellieni, C. (2010). Neonatal pain and oxidative stress. *Minerva Pediatrica 62*(Supplement 1), 59-60.

Carbaugh, S.F. (2004). Understanding shaken baby syndrome. *Advances in Neonatal Care, 4*, 105-114.

Carlton, P., Johnson, I., & Cunliffe, C. (2009). Factors influencing parents' decision to choose chiropractic care for their children in the UK. *Clinical Chiropractic, 12*, 11-22.

Casaer, P. (1979). Postural behaviour in newborn infants. *Clinic in Developmental Medicine Number 72*. London: William Heinemann Medical Books.

Cheng, J.C., & Au, A.W. (1994). Infantile torticollis: A review of 624 cases. *Journal Pediatric Orthopedics, 14*(6), 802-808.

Chen, M.M., Chang, H.S., Hsieh, C.F., Yen, M.F., & Chen, T.H. (2005). Predictive model for congenital muscular torticollis: Analysis of 1021 infants with sonography. *Archives Physical Medical Rehabilitation, 86*(11), 2199-2203.

Chez, R.A., & Spellacy, W.N. (1994). Fractured clavicle is an unavoidable event. *American Journal of Obstetrics & Gynecology, 171*, 797-798.

Cioni, G., Ferrari, F., & Prechtl, H.F.R. (1989). Posture and spontaneous motility in full-term infants. *Early Human Development 18*, 247-262.

Cincotta, D.R., Crawford, N.W., Lim, A., Cranswick, N.E., Skull, S., South, M., & Powell, C.V. (2006). Comparison of complementary and alternative medicine use: reasons and motivations between two tertiary children's hospitals. *Archives of Disease in Childhood, 91*(2), 153-158.

Colloca, C., Keller, T.S., & Gunzburg, R. (2004). Biomechanical and neurophysiological responses to spinal manipulation in patients with lumbar radiculopathy. *Journal of Manipulative and Physiological Therapeutics, 27*(1), 1-15.

Conroy, S.M., Choonara, I., Impicciatore, P., Mohn, A., Arnel, H., Rane, A., Knoeppels, C., Seyberth, H., Pandolfina, C., & Raffaelli, M.P. (2000). Survey of unlicensed and off-label drug use in paediatric wards in European countries. *BMJ, 320*, 79-82.

Crouch, J.L., Skowronski, J.J., Milner, J.S., & Harris, B. (2008). Parental response to infant crying: The influence of child physical abuse risk and hostile priming. *Child Abuse and Neglect, 32*, 702-710.

Dobson, D., Lucassen, P.L.B.J., Miller, J.E., Vlieger, A.M., Prescott, P., & Lewith, G. (2012). *Manipulative therapies for infantile colic*. Cochrane Database of Systematic Reviews 2012, Issue 12. Art. No.: CD004796. DOI: 10.1002/14651858.CD004796.pub2.

Dorlands Medical Dictionary, 26th edition. (1991). London: WB Saunders Company.

Dorland's Illustrated Medical Dictionary, 31st Ed. (2007). Philadelphia: WB Saunders, p.389(ch 11)

Douglas, P., & Hill, P. (2011). Managing infants who cry excessively in the first few months of life. *British Medical Journal, 343*, d7772.

Edwards, D., Gibb, C., & Cook, J. (2010). The benefits of chiropractic intervention for babies with sleep deprivation resulting from birth trauma. *Midwifery Digest, 20*(3), 373-379.

Engel, G.L. (1977). The need for a new medical model: A challenge for biomedicine. *Science, 196*, 129–136.

Ernst, E. (2009). Chiropractic spinal manipulation for infant colic: A systematic review of randomized trials. *International Journal of Clinical Practice, 63*(9), 1351-1353.

Farber, S.D. (1982). *Neurorehabilitation: A multi-sensory approach.* Philadelphia: W. B. Saunders

Faure, M., & Richardson, A. (2008). *Baby sense.* Welgemoed, South Africa: Metz Press.

Fava, G.A., & Sonino, N. (2008). The biopsychosocial model thirty years later. *Psychotherapy Psychosomatics, 77*, 1-2.

Ferreira, J.H., & James, J.I.P. (1972). Progressive and resolving infantile idiopathic scoliosis: The differential diagnosis. *Journal Bone and Joint Surgery of America, 54-B*, 648-655.

Field, T., Diego, M., Cullen, C., Hernandez-Reif, M., Sunshine, W., & Douglas, S. (2002). Fibromyalgia pain and substance P decrease and sleep improves after massage therapy. *Journal Clinical Rheumatology, 8*, 72-76.

Field, T. (2002). Massage therapy. *Medical Clinics of North America, 86*, 283-313.

Finley, A.G., Franck, L.S., Grunau, R., & von Baeyer, C.L. (2005). Why children's pain matters. *International Association for the Study of Pain Task Force on Acute Pain, XIII*(4), 1-2.

Fischer, D., Stewart, A.L., Bloch, D.A., Lorig, K., Laurent, D., & Holman, H. (1999). Capturing the patient's view of change as a clinical outcome measure. *Journal American Medical Association, 282*(12), 1157-1162.

Fitzgerald, M., & Beggs, S. (2001). The neurobiology of pain: Developmental aspects. *Neuroscientist, 7*, 246-257.

Fitzgerald, M., & Walker, S. (2009). Infant pain management: A developmental neurobiological approach. *Nature Clinical Practical Neurology, 5*, 35-50.

Foster, N.E., Hartvigsen, J., & Croft, P. (2012). Taking responsibility for the early assessment and treatment of patients with musculoskeletal pain: A review and critical analysis. *Arthritis Research and Therapy, 14*(205), 1-9.

Freedman, S.B., Al-Harthy, N., & Thull-Freedman, J. (2009). The crying infant: Diagnostic testing and frequency of serious underlying disease. *Pediatrics, 123*(3), 841-848.

Frymann, V. (1966). Relation of disturbances of craniosacral mechanisms to symptomatology of the newborn: Study of 1250 infants. *Journal American Osteopathic Association, 65*, 1059-1075.

Garrison, M.M., & Christakis, D.A. (2000). Early childhood: Colic, child development and poisoning prevention. A systematic review of treatments for infant colic. *Pediatrics, 106*, 184-190.

Geertsma, M.A., & Hyams, J.S. (1989). Colic—a pain syndrome of infancy? *Pediatric Clinics of North America, 36*(4), 288-293.

General Chiropractic Council. (2010). *Code of Practice and Standard of Proficiency, 4th Edition* (p. 5). Effective from 30 June 2010. London: Author.

Gill, I., & Sharif, F. (2012). A disjointed effort: Paediatric musculoskeletal examination. *Archives of Disease in Childhood, 97*, 641-643.

Gorlia, T., van den Bent, M.J., Hegi, M.E., Mirimanof, R.O., Weller, M., & Cairncross, J.C., (2008). Nomograms for predicting survival of patients with newly diagnosed glioblastoma: Prognostic factor analysis of EORTC and NCIC trial 26981-22982/CE.3. *Lancet Oncology, 9*(1), 29-38.

Gottlieb, M.S. (1993). Neglected spinal cord, brain stem and musculoskeletal injuries stemming from birth trauma. *JMPT, 16*(8), 537-543.

Gudmundsson, G. (2010). Infantile colic: Is a pain syndrome. *Medical Hypothesis, 75*, 528-529.

Guyatt, G. (2016). Dave Sackett and the ethos of the EBM community. *Journal Clinical Epidemiology, 73*, 75-78.

Hagh, L. (2005). *Retrospective study into long-term effects of infantile colic on sleep and behaviour of 2-3-year-olds.* Project Report. Bournemouth, UK: Anglo-European College of Chiropractic.

Hall, R.T., Mercer, A.M., Teasley, S.L., McPherson, D.M., Simon, S.D., Santos, S.R., Meyers, B.M., & Hipsh, N.E. (2002). A breast-feeding assessment score to evaluate the risk for cessation of breast-feeding by 7-10 days of age. *Journal of Pediatrics, 141*(5), 659-664.

Hall, B., Chesters, J., & Robinson, A. (2011). Infantile colic: A systematic review of medical and conventional therapies. *Journal of Paediatrics and Child Health, 48*(2), 128-137.

Hanson, H.A., & Miller, J.E. (2018). An electronic parent reported infant outcomes measure in chiropractic clinics: A feasibility study. *Journal Clinical Chiropractic Pediatrics, 17*(1), 1413-1417.

Hawk, C., Schneider, M., Ferrance, R., Hewitt, E., Van Loon, M., & Tanis L. (2009). Best practices recommendations for chiropractic care of infants, children and adolescents: Results of a consensus process. *Journal of Manipulative and Physiological Therapeutics, 32,* 639-647.

Hawk, C., Shneider, M.J., Vallone, S., & Hewitt, E.G. (2016). Best practices recommendations for chiropractic care of children: A consensus update. *Journal of Manipulative and Physiological Therapeutics, 39*(3), 158-168. Accessed August 21,2016: http://www.ncbi.nlm.nih.gov/pubmed/27040034 .

Hayden, C., & Mullinger, B. (2006). A preliminary assessment of the impact of cranial osteopathy for the relief of infant colic. *Complementary Therapies in Clinical Practice, 12,* 83-90.

Hemmi, M.H., Wolke, D.,, & Schneider, S. (2011). Associations between problems with crying, sleeping and/or feeding in infancy and long-term behavioural outcomes in childhood: A meta-analysis. *Archives of Diseases in Childhood, 96,* 622-629.

Hermann, C., Hobmeister, J., Demirakca, S., Zohsel, K., & Flor, H. (2006) Long-term alteration of pain sensitivity in school-aged children with early pain experiences. *Pain, 125,* 278-285.

Herzaft-LeRoy, J., Xhignesse, M., & Gaboury, I. (2017). Efficacy of an osteopathic treatment coupled with lactation consultant for infants' biomechanical sucking difficulties. *Journal of Human Lactation, 33*(1), 165-172.

Hestbaek, L., Jorgensen, A., & Hartvigsen, J. (2009). A description of children and adolescents in Danish chiropractic practice: Results from a nationwide survey. *Journal of Manipulative and Physiologic Therapy, 32*(8), 607-615.

Hiew, M., Kwong, D.S., Mok, Z., Tee, Y.H., & Miller, J.E. (2018). Portable pad or pen and paper? Preference of mothers completing an outcomes instrument: A cross-sectional survey. *Journal Clinical Chiropractic Pediatrics, 17*(2), 1441-1443.

Hipperson, A.J. (2004). Chiropractic management of infantile colic. *Clinical Chiropractic, 7,* 180-186.

Hirji, K.F., & Fagerland, M.W. (2009). Outcome-based subgroups analysis: A neglected concern. *Trials, 10,* 33. doi: 10.1186/1745-6215-10-33

Hogdall, C.K., Vestermark, V., Birch, M., Plenov, G., & Toftager-Larsen, K. (1991). The significance of pregnancy and postpartum factors for the development of infant colic. *Journal Perinatal Medicine, 19,* 251-257.

Holmes, E., & Miller, J. (2014). Adverse reactions of medications in children: The need for vigilance, a case study. *Journal of Clinical Chiropractic Pediatrics, 14*(2), www.jcccponline.com

Homdrom, A.K.S., & Miller, J.E. (2015). Maternal report of feeding practices: A cross-sectional survey of 1753 mother presenting infants to a chiropractic teaching clinic. *Journal of Clinical Chiropractic Pediatrics, 15*(1), 1198-1202.

Hon, K-LE., Kam, W-YC., Leung, T-F., Lam, M-CA., Wong, K-Y., Lee, K-CK., Luk, N-MT., Fox, T-F., & Ng, P-C. (2006). Steroid fears in children with eczema. *Acta Paediatrica, 95*(11), 1451-1455.

Honda, N., Ohgi, S., Wada, N., Loo, K.K., Hagashimoto, Y., & Fukuda K. (2013). Effect of therapeutic touch on brain activation of preterm infants in response to sensory punctate stimulus: A near-infrared spectropscopy-based study. *ADC Fetal and Neonatal Edition, 98*(3), F244-F249.

Howard, C.R., Lanphear, N., Lanphear, B.P., Eberly, S., & Lawrence, R.A. (2006). Parental responses to infant crying and colic: The effect on breastfeeding duration. *Breastfeeding Medicine, 1*(3), 146-155.

Hughes, S., & Bolton, J. (2002). Is chiropractic an effective treatment in infantile colic? *Archives of Disease in Childhood, 86*, 382-384.

Humphreys, B.K. (2010). Possible adverse events in children treated by manual therapy: A review. *Chiropractic & Osteopathy, 18*, 12. doi: 10.1186/1746-1340-18-12]

Illingsworth, R. (1985). Infantile colic revisited. *Archives of Disease in Childhood, 60*, 981-985.

Ip, S., Chung, M., Raman, G., Trikalinos, T.A., & Lau, J. (2009). A summary of the Agency for Healthcare Research and Quality's evidence report on breastfeeding in developed countries. *Breastfeeding Medicine, 4* (suppl 1), S17-S30.

Jandial, S., Myers, A., & Wise, E. (2009). Doctors likely to encounter children with musculoskeletal complaints have low confidence in their clinical skills. *Journal Pediatrics, 154*, 267-271.

Jaskulski, J., & Miller, J. (2018). Infant demographic profile and parent report of treatment outcomes at chiropractic clinic in the UK: An observational study. *Journal Clinical Chiropractic Pediatrics, 17*(1), 1398-1404.

Johnston, C.C., & von Baeyer, C.L. (2012). A measure of pediatric pain intensity across ages and clinical conditions. *Pain, 153*, 1545-1546.

Joseph, P., & Rosenfeld, W. (1990). Clavicular fractures in neonates. *Archives Pediatric and Adolescent Medicine, 144*(2), 165-167.

Karpelowsky, A.S. (2004). *The efficacy of chiropractic spinal manipulative therapy in the treatment of infantile colic.* MSc Dissertation. Health Sciences, Technikon Witwatersrand. Johannesburg, South Africa.

Katkade, V.B., Sanders, K.K.N., & Sou, K.H. (2018). Real world data: An opportunity to supplement existing evidence for the use of long-established medicines in health care decision-making. *Journal of Multidiscplinary Healthcare, 11,* 295-304.

Kemper, K.J., Vohra, S., & Walls, R. (2008). The Task Force on Complementary and Alternative Medicine, the Provisional Section on Complementary, Holistic and Integrative Medicine. The use of complementary and alternative medicine in paediatrics. *Pediatrics, 122*(6), 1374-1386.

Klougart, N., Nilsson, N., & Jacobs, J. (1989). Infantile colic treated by chiropractors: A prospective study of 316 cases. *Journal of Manipulative and Physiological Therapeutics, 12,* 281-288.

Koch, L.E., Koch, H., Graumann-Brunt, S., Stolle, D., Ramirez, J.-M., & Saternus, K.S. (2002). Heart rate changes in response to mild mechanical irritation of the high cervical spinal cord region in infants. *Forensic Science International, 128,* 168-176.

Koonin, S.D., Karpelowsky, A.S., Yelverton, C.J., & Rubens, B.N. (2002). *A comparative study to determine the efficacy of chiropractic spinal manipulative therapy and allopathic medication in the treatment of infantile colic* [abstract] (p. 18). World Federation of Chiropractic 7th Biennial Congress. Orlando (FL): World Federation of Chiropractic.

Kozak, L.J., & Weeks, J.D. (2002). U.S. Trends in obstetrics procedures, 1990-2000. *Birth, 29*(3), 157-161.

Kvitvaeer, B., Miller, J., & Newell, D. (2010). Improving our understanding of the irritable infant: An observational study in a chiropractic teaching clinic. *Journal Clinical Nursing, 21,* 63-69.

LaGasse, L.L., Neal, A.R., & Lester, B.M. (2008). Infantile colic: Acoustic cry characteristics, maternal perception of cry, and temperament. *Mental Retardation and Developmental Disabilities Research Reviews, 11,* 83-95.

Levine, M.G., Holroyde, J., Woods, J.R., Siddiqi, T.A., Scott, M., Miodovnik, M. et al. (1984). Birth trauma: Incidence and predisposing factors. *Obstetrics and Gynecology, 63*(6), 792-795.

Lidow, M.S. (2002). Long-term effects of neonatal pain on nociceptive systems. *Pain, 99,* 377-383.

Lucassen, P. (2010). Colic in infants. *Clinical Evidence, 02,* 309.

Lundqvist, P., Hellstrom-Westas, L., & Hallstrom, I. (2014). Reorganizing life. A qualitative study of father's lived experience in the 3 years subsequent to the very preterm birth of their child. *Journal of Pediatric Nursing: Nursing Care of Children and Families, 29*(2), 124-131.

Marchand, A. (2013). A proposed model with possible implications for safety and technique adaptations for chiropractic spinal manipulative therapy for infants and children. *Journal Manipulative and Physiological Therapeutics, 5,* 1-14.

Marrilier, K.E., Lima, A.M., Donovan L.Y., Taylor, C., & Miller, J. (2014). Mama please stop crying; lowered post-natal depression scores in mothers after a course of chiropractic care for their infants. *Journal Clinical Chiropractic Pediatrics, 14*(3), 1179-1182.

Martin-Du Pau, R.C., Benoit, R., & Girardier, L. (2004). The role of body position and gravity in the symptoms and treatment of various medical diseases. *Swiss Medical Weekly, 134,* 543-551.

Mavrogenis, A.F., Mitsiokapa, E.A., Kanellopoulos, A.D., Ruggieri, P., & Papagelopoulos, P.J. (2011). Birth fracture of the clavicle. *Advanced Neonatal Care, 11*(5), 328-341.

McCann, L.J., & Newell, S.J. (2006). Survey of pediatric complementary and alternative medicine in health and chronic disease. *Archives of Diseases of Childhood, 91,* 173-174.

McGhee, J.L., Burks, F.N., Sheckels, J.L., & Jarvis, J.N. (2002). Identifying children with chronic arthritis based chief complaints: Absence of predictive value for musculoskeletal pain as an indicator of rheumatic disease in children. *Pediatrics, 110*(2), 354-359.

Mercer, C., & Nook, B.C. (1999). The efficacy of chiropractic spinal adjustments as a treatment protocol in the management of infantile colic. In S.Haldeman, & B. Murphy, Eds., *5th Biennial Congress of the World Federation of Chiropractic* (pp. 170-171). Auckland, New Zealand WFC.

Miller, A., & Barr, R. (1991). Infantile colic. Is it a gut issue? *Pediatric Clinics of North America, 38*(6), 1407-1423.

Miller, J., & Caprini Croci, S. (2005). Cry baby, why baby? Beyond colic: Is it time to widen our views? *Journal Clinical Chiropractic Pediatrics, 6*(3), 419-423.

Miller, J., Hanson, H., Hiew, M., Kwong, D. S., Mok, Z., & Tee, Y.H. (in press). Maternal report of outcomes of chiropractic care for infants. *Journal Manipulative and Physiological Therapeutics.*

Miller, J. (2010). Demographic survey of pediatric patients presenting to a chiropractic teaching clinic. *Chiropractic & Osteopathy, 18,* 33.

Miller, R.I., & Clarrens, S.K. (2000). Long-term developmental outcomes in patients with deformational plagiocephaly. *Pediatrics, 105*(2), 1-5.

Miller, J., Beharie, M., Taylor, A., Simmenes E.B., & Way S. (2016). Parent reports of exclusive breastfeeding after attending a combined midwifery and chiropractic feeding clinic in the United Kingdom: A cross-sectional service evaluation. *Journal of Evidence Based Alternative and Complementary Medicine, 21(2),* 1-7. DOI: 10.1177/2156587215625399

Miller, J.E., & Benfield, K. (2008). Adverse effects of spinal manipulative therapy in children younger than 3 years: A retrospective study in a chiropractic teaching clinic. *Journal Manipulative and Physiological Therapeutics, 31*(6), 419-423.

Miller, J., Miller, L., Sulesund, A-K., & Yevtushenko A. (2009). Contribution of chiropractic therapy to resolving suboptimal breastfeeding: A case series of 114 infants. *Journal of Manipulative and Physiological Therapeutics, 32*(8), 670-674.

Miller, J., & Phillips, H. (2009). Long-term effects of infant colic: A survey comparison of chiropractic treatments and non-treatment groups. *Journal of Manipulative and Physiological Therapeutics, 32*(8), 635-638.

Miller, J., & Newell, D. (2012). Prognostic significance of subgroup classification of infant patients with crying disorders: A prospective cohort study. *Journal Canadian Chiropractic Association, 56*(1), 40-48.

Miller, J., Newell, D., & Bolton, J. (2012). Efficacy of chiropractic manual therapy in infant colic: A pragmatic single-blind, randomised controlled trial. *Journal of Manipulative and Physiological Therapeutics, 35*(8), 600-607.

Miller, J., Newell, D., & Bolton, J. (2012). Efficacy of chiropractic manual therapy in infant colic: A pragmatic single-blind, randomized controlled trial. *Archives of Disease Childhood, 97*(supplement 1), 114.

Miller, J.E. (2013). Costs of routine care for infant colic in the UK and costs of chiropractic manual therapy as a management strategy alongside a RCT for this condition. *Journal of Clinical and Chiropractic Pediatrics, 14*(1), 1063-1069.

Miller, A., Telford, A., Huizinga, B., Pinkster, M., Telford, A.C.J., & ten Heggeler, J.M., & Miller, J.E. et al. (2015). What breastfeeding mothers want. *Clinical Lactation, 6*(3), 117-121.

Miller, J., & Weber-Hellstenius S., (2013). Is infant colic an allergic response to cow's milk? What is the evidence? *Journal of Clinical Chiropractic Pediatrics, 14*(1), 1097-1102.

Miller, J., Miller, A.S., Huizinga, B., Pinkster, M., Telford, A.C.J., & ten Heggeler, J.M. (2016). Development and testing of a multidimensional parent reported outcome measure for common presenting complaint of infancy: The UK Infant Questionnaire. *Journal of Clinical Chiropractic Pediatrics, 15*(3), 1292-1300.

Minns, R.A., Jones, P., & Mok, J.Y.Q. (2008). Incidence and demography of non-accidental head injury in southeast Scotland from a national database. *American Journal of Preventive Medicine, 34*(4S), 126-133.

Monson, T. (2013, March 26). Personal communication.

Mootz, R.D., Hansen, D.T., Breen, A., Killinger, L.Z., & Nelson, C. (2006). Health services research related to chiropractic: Review and recommendations for research prioritization by the chiropractic profession. *Journal of Manipulative and Physiological Therapeutics, 29*(9), 707-725.

Morris, S., St James-Robert, I., Sleep, J., & Gillham, P. (2001). Economic evaluation of strategies for managing crying and sleeping problems. *Archives of Disease in Childhood, 84,* 15-19.

Moyer, C.A., Rounds, J., & Hannum, J.W. (2004). A meta-analysis of massage therapy research. *Psychological Bulletin, 130,* 3-18.

Murphy, D., & Hurwitz, E. (2007). A theoretical model for the development of a diagnosis-based clinic decision rule for the management of patients with spinal pain. *BMC Musculoskeletal Disorders, 8,* 75-86.

Murphy, D.R., Justice, B.D., Paskowski, I.C., Perle, S.M., & Schneider, M.J. (2011). The establishment of a primary spine care practitioner and its benefits to health care reform. *Chiropractic and Manual Therapies, 19,* 17.

Murray, A.D. (1979). Infant crying as an elicitor of parental behaviour: An examination of two models. *Psychological Bulletin, 86,* 191-215.

National Center for Alternative and Complementary Medicine. (2007). Retrieved from http://www.nccamnih.gov.

National Health Service. (2015). *Patient reported outcome measures (PROMS).* Retrieved from https:www.england.nhs/uk/statistics statistical work-areas-proms. 2015

Nyiendo. J., Haas, M., & Hondras, M.A. (1997). Outcomes research in chiropractic: The state of the art and recommendations for the chiropractic research agenda. *Journal Manipulative and Physiologic Therapeutics, 20*(3), 185-200.

Olafsdottir, E., Forshei, S., Fluge, G., & Markestad, T. (2001). Randomized controlled trial of infant colic treated with chiropractic spinal manipulation. *Archives of Disease in Childhood, 84*, 138-141.

Papousek, M., & von Hofacker, N. (1998). Persistent crying in early infancy: A non-trivial condition of risk for the developing mother-infant relationship. *Child Care Health and Development, 5*, 395-424.

Parker, L.A. (2005). Early recognition and treatment of birth trauma: Injuries to the head and face. *Advances in Neonatal Care, 5*(6), 288-297.

Philippi, H., Faldum, A., Schleupen, A., Pabst, B., Jung, T., Bergmann, H., Bieber, I., Kaemmerer, C., Dijs, P., & Reitter, B. (2006). Infantile posture asymmetry and osteopathic treatment: A randomized therapeutic trial. *Developmental Medicine and Child Neurology, 48*, 5-9.

Prechtl, H.F.R., Einspeiler, C., Cioni, G., Bos, A.F., Ferrari, F., & Sontheimer, D. (1997). An early marker for neurological deficits after perinatal brain lesions. *Lancet, 349*, 1361-1363.

Rao, M., Brenner, R., Schisterman, E., Vik, T., & Mills, J. (2004). Long-term cognitive development in children with prolonged crying. *Archives of Disease in Childhood, 89*, 989-992.

Rabelo, N.N., Matushita, H., & Cardeal, D.D., (2017). Traumatic brain lesions in newborns. *Arq Neurosiquitr, 75(3), 180-188.*

Rautava, P., Lehtonen, L., Helenius, H., & Sillanpaa, M. (1995). Infantile colic: Child and family three years later. *Pediatrics, 96*(1), 43-47.

Reher, C., Kuny, K.D., Pantalitschka, T., Urschitz, M.S., & Poets, C.F. (2008). Randomised crossover trial of different postural interventions on bradycardia and intermittent hypoxia in preterm infants. *Archives Disease of Childhood Foetal Neonatal Education, 93*, F289-F291.

Reijneveld, S.A., van der Wal, M.F., Brugman, E., & Hira Sing, R.A., & Verloove-Vanhorick, S.P. (2004). Infant crying and abuse. *Lancet, 364*, 1340-1342.

Ritzman, D. (2004). Birthing interventions and the newborn cervical spine. In H. Biedermann (Ed.), *Manual therapy in children* (pp. 75-81). Edinburgh: Churchill Livingstone.

Romanello, S., Spiri, D., Marcuzzi, E., Zanin, A., Boizeau, P., Riviere, S., Vizeneux, A., Moretti, R., Carbajal, R., Mercier, J.C., Wood, C., Zuccotti, V., Crichiutti, G., Alerberti, C., & Titomanlio, L. (2013).

Association between childhood migraine and history of infantile colic. *Journal American Medical Association, 309*(15), 1607-1612.

Rosenbaum, P. (2006). Commentary on infantile posture asymmetry and osteopathic treatment: A randomized therapeutic trial. *Developmental Medicine and Child Neurology, 48*, 4.

Rossitch, E., & Oakes, W.J. (1992). Perinatal spinal cord injury: Clinical, radiographic and pathologic features. *Pediatric Neurosurgery, 18*, 149-152

Sanson, A., Prior, M., & Oberklaid, F. (1985). Normative data on temperament in Australian infants. *Australian Journal of Psychology, 37*, 185-195.

Savino, F., Castagno, E., Bretto, R., Brondello, C., Palumeri, E., & Oggero R. (2005). A prospective 10-year study of children who had severe infantile colic. *Acta Paeditrica Supplement, 94*(449), 129-132.

Schmid, P.H., Hetlevik, M.A., & Miller, J. (2016). Infant presentations and outcomes at a chiropractic clinic in the UK: Parent report of treatment outcomes using United Kingdom Infant Questionnaire (UKIQ). *Journal Clinical Chiropractic Pediatrics, 15*(2), 1237-1242.

Scott, P.E., & Campbell, G. (1998). Interpretation of subgroup analyses in medical device clinical trials. *Drug Information Journal, 32*, 213-220.

Seaman, D.R., & Cleveland, C. (1999). Spinal pain syndromes: Nociceptive, neuropathic and psychologic mechanisms. *Journal of Manipulative and Physiological Therapeutics, 22*(7), 458-472.

Shafir, Y., & Kaufman, B.A. (1992). Quadraplegia after chiropractic manipulation in an infant with congenital torticollis caused by a spinal cord astrocytoma. *Journal of Pediatrics, 120*(2), 266-269.

Sival, D.A., Prechtl, H.F.R., Sonder, G.H.A., & Touwen, B.C.L. (1993). The effect of intrauterine breech position on postnatal motor function of the lower limbs. *Early Human Development, 32*, 161-176.

Sharfstein, J.M., North, M., & Serwint, J.R. (2007). Over the counter but no longer under the radar: Pediatric cough and cold medications. *New England Journal of Medicine, 357*(23), 2321-2324.

Slaven, E.J., & Mathers, J. (2010). Differential diagnosis of shoulder and cervical pain: A case report. *Journal of Manual and Manipulative Therapy, 18*(4), 191-196.

Smith, L.J. (2007). Impact of birthing practices on the breastfeeding dyad. *Journal of Midwifery and Women's Health, 52*(6), 621-630.

Smith, L.L., Keating, M.N., Holbert, D., Spratt, D.J., McCammon, M.R., Smith, S.S., & Isreal, R.G. (1994). The effects of athletic massage on delayed onset muscle soreness, creatine kinase and neutrophil count: A preliminary report. *Journal Orthopedic Sports Physical Therapy, 19,* 93-99.

South, M., & Lim, A. (2003). Use of complementary and alternative medicine in children: Too important to ignore. *Journal Paediatrics and Child Health, 39,* 573-574.

St. James-Roberts, I., & Halil, T. (1991). Infant crying patterns in the first year: Normal community and clinical findings. *Journal of Child Psychology and Psychiatry, 32*(6), 951-968.

St James-Roberts, I., Hurry, J., Bowyer, J., & Barr, R.G. (1995). Supplementary carrying compared with advice to increase responsive parenting as interventions to prevent persistent infant crying. *Pediatrics, 95*(3), 381-388.

St. James-Roberts, I. (1990). What is distinct about infants' colic cries? *Archives of Disease of Childhood, 80,* 56-62.

St. James-Roberts, I., Sleep, J., Morris, S., Owen, C., & Gillham, P. (2001). Use of a behavioural programme in the first 3 months to prevent infant crying and sleeping problems. *Journal of Paediatrics and Child Health, 37,* 289-297.

St. James-Roberts, I. (2008). Infant crying and sleeping: Helping parents to prevent and manage problems. *Primary Care: Clinics in Office Practice, 35*(3), 547-567.

Stellwagen, L., Hubbard, E., Chambers, C., & Lyons Jones, K. (2008). Torticollis, facial asymmetry and plagiocephaly in normal newborns. *Archives of Disease in Childhood, 93*(10), 827-831.

Stephenson, T.J. (2005). The National Patient Safety Agency. *Archives of Diseases of Childhood, 90,* 226-228.

Taylor, A., Atkins, R., Kumar, R., Adams, D., & Glover, V. (2005). A new Mother-to-Infant Bonding Scale: Links with early maternal mood. *Archives of Women's Mental Health, 8,* 45-51.

Thiel, H., & Bolton, J. (2006). The reporting of patient safety incidents—first experiences with the chiropractic reporting and learning system (CRLS): A pilot study. *Clinical Chiropractic, 9,* 139-149.

Todd, A.J., Carroll, M.T., Robinson, A., & Mitchell, E.K. (2015). Adverse events due to chiropractic and other manual therapies for infants and children: A review of literature. *Journal Manipulative Physiological Therapeutics, 38*(9), 699-712.

Torvaldsen, S., Roberts, C.L., Simpson, J.M., Thompson, J.F., & Ellwood, D.A. (2006). Intrapartum epidural analgesia and breastfeeding: A prospective cohort study. *International Breastfeeding Journal, 1*, 24.

Tow, J., & Vallone, S. (2009). Development of an integrative relationship in the care of the breastfeeding newborn: Lactation consultant and chiropractor. *Journal Clinical Chiropractic Pediatrics, 10*, 626-632.

Towbin, A. (1964). Spinal cord and brainstem injury at birth. *Archives of Pathology, 77*, 620-632.

Van Rijn, R.R., Bilo, R.A.C., & Robben, S.G.F. (2009). Birth-related mid-posterior rib fractures in neonates: A report of three cases (and a possible fourth case) and a review of the literature. *Pediatric Radiology, 39*, 30-34.

Vernacchio, L., Kelly, J.P., Kaufman, D.W., & Mitchell, A.A. (2009). Medication use among children <12 years of age in the United States: Results from the Slone survey. *Pediatrics, 124*(2), 446-454.

Victora, C.F., Bahl, Barros, A.J.D., Franca, G.V., Horton, S., Krasevec J. et.al., (2016). Breastfeeding in the 21st century: epidemiology, mechanisms and lifelong effect. *The Lancet, 387*(10017), 475-490.

Vik, T., Grote, V., Escribano, J., Socha, J., Verduci, E., Fritsch, M., Carlier, C., von Kries, R., & Koletzko, B. (2009). Infantile colic, prolonged crying and maternal postnatal depression. *Acta Paediatrica, 98*, 1344-1348.

Vohra, S., Johnston, B.C., Cramer, K., & Humphreys, K. (2007). Adverse events associated with pediatric spinal manipulation: A systematic review. *Pediatrics, 119*(1), e275-283.

Von Kries, R., Kalies, H., & Papousek, M. (2006). Excessive crying beyond 3 months may herald other features of multiple regulatory problems. *Archives Pediatric and Adolescent Medicine, 160*, 508-511.

Walker, S.M., Tochiki, K.K., & Fitzgerald, M. (2009). Hind-paw incision in early life increases the hyperalgesic response to repeat surgical injury: Critical period and dependence on initial afferent activity. *Pain, 147*, 99-106.

Wall, V., & Glass, R. (2006). Mandibular asymmetry and breastfeeding problems: Experience from 11 cases. *Journal of Human Lactation, 22*(3), 328-334.

Wessel, M.A., Cobb, J.C., Jackson, E.B., Harris, G.S., & Detwilter, B.A. (1954). Paroxysmal fussing in infancy, sometimes called "colic." *Pediatrics, 14*(5), 421-433.

Wiberg, K.R., & Wiberg, J.M. (2010). A retrospective study of chiropractic treatment of 276 Danish infants with infantile colic. *Journal Manipulative and Physiological Therapeutics, 33*, 536-541.

Wiberg, J.M.M., Nordsteen, J., & Nilsson, N. (1999). The short-term effect of spinal manipulation in the treatment of infantile colic: A randomized controlled clinical trial with a blinded observer. *Journal Manipulative and Physiological Therapeutics, 22,* 517-22.

Williams-Frey, S. (2011). Management of atypical infant colic – A pain syndrome of infancy - and the emotional stress associated with it. Why treat a benign disorder? *Clinical Chiropractic, 14,* 91-96.

Wirtz, S.J., & Trent, R.B. (2008). Passive surveillance of shaken-baby syndrome using hospital inpatient data. *American Journal of Preventive Medicine, 34*(4S), 134-139.

Wolke, D., Rizzo, P., & Woods, S. (2002). Persistent infant crying and hyperactivity problems in middle childhood. *Pediatrics, 109*(6), 1054-1060.

World Health Organization. (2005). *Guidelines on chiropractic.* Geneva, Switzerland: WHO Press. Retrieved from http:www.WHO/int/whv/2010/10_summary_en_pdf.

World Health Organization. (2012). *Guidelines on basic training and safety in chiropractic.* Geneva, Switzerland: WHO Press.

World Health Organization.(2012). *Bone and joint press release: Global burden of musculoskeletal diseases.* Retrieved from www.WHO.int/topics/ healthrisks_mortality

Wright, C., Beard, H., Cox, J., Scott, P., & Miller, J. (2014). Parents' choice of non-supine sleep position for newborns: A cross-sectional study. *British Journal of Midwifery, 22*(9), 625-629.

Yalcin, S.S., Orun, E., Mutlu, B., Madendag, Y., Sinici, I., Dursun, A., Ozkara, H.A., Ustunyurt, Z., Kutluk, S., & Yurdakok, K. (2010). Why are they having colic? A nested case-control study. *Paediatric and Perinatal Epidemiology, 24,*.584-596.

Zimmerman, A.W., Kumar, A.J., Gadoth, N., & Hodges, F.J., 3rd. (1978). Traumatic vertebrobasilar occlusive disease in childhood. *Neurology, 28,* 185-188.

Zuzak, T.J., Boňková, J., Caredduc, D., Garamid, M., Hadjipanayise, A., Jazbec, J., Merrick, J., & Miller, J. (2012). Published data and expert perspectives on the use of complementary and alternative medicine by children in Europe. *Journal Alternative and Complementary Therapies in Medicine, 21*(suppl 1), S34-47. doi:10.1016/j.ctim.2012.01.001

Zwart, P., Vellema-Goud, M.G.A., & Brand, P.L.P.(2007). Characteristics of infants admitted to hospital for persistent colic and comparison with healthy infants. *Acta Paediatrica, 96,* 401-405.

Made in the USA
Columbia, SC
01 June 2022

61145508R00080